Cook, Ann

Professed Cookery

ISBN: 978-1-948837-19-4

This classic reprint was produced from digital files in the Google Books digital collection, which may be found at http://www.books.google.com. The artwork used on the cover is from Wikimedia Commons and remains in the public domain. Omissions and/or errors in this book are due to either the physical condition of the original book or due to the scanning process by Google or its agents.

This edition of Ann Cook's **Professed Cookery** was originally published in 1760 (London).

Townsends
PO Box 415, Pierceton, IN 46562
www.Townsends.us

PROFESSED
COOKERY:

CONTAINING

BOILING,	PICKLING,
ROASTING,	POTTING,
PASTRY,	MADE-WINES,
PRESERVING,	GELLIES,

And Part of CONFECTIONARIES.

With an ESSAY upon the

LADY's ART of COOKERY:

TOGETHER WITH
A PLAN of HOUSE-KEEPING.

By ANN COOK,

Teacher of the True ART of COOKERY.

The THIRD EDITION.

LONDON:

Printed for and fold by the AUTHOR, at her Lodgings,
in Mr. MOOR's, Cabinet-maker, FULLER's RENTS,
HOLBORN. Price Six Shillings.

To the READER.

IF long Experience make all Fools wife,
  It will enable me to criticize;
A poor Mind, if known, might be conceal'd,
Mean Poverty is fhewn when its reveal'd.
A Lady claims fuch Skill in dreffing Meat,
Prefcribes to Lords and Ladies what to eat;
From what fhe does collect makes up a Book,
Affumes the Author and the fov'reign Cook,
Of fo much Art, that each ignorant Maid
By reading it, is Miftrefs of the Trade;
Shall know to do the Art of Cook'ry well,
Examines not for Judgment, Tafte or Smell.
Look and behold the Lady's Introduction,
Her noble Progrefs promis'd by Inftruction,
The lower Sort makes Choice of, for to fway, ⎫
And fays, will treat them in their own Way, ⎬
For fuch a Teacher's Reformation pray: ⎭

To fleece the poor low Servants to get Wealth,
And collect Surfeits to deftroy all Health,
Can this be honefty or pelf'ring Stealth;
Robbers on the Highway may take a Purfe,
But who fteals away Health is ten Times worfe,
Good Cooks are Bleffings and bad Cooks a Curfe.
Th' Cook'ry Art got Birthright and a Bleffing,
Which all true *Ifra'lites* are ftill poffeffing;
Jacob's good Broth, *Rebecca*'s fav'ry Meat,
Sets forth the Worth of Cooks that are compleat.
She fteals from ev'ry Author to her Book,
Infamoufly branding the pillag'd Cook,
With Trick, Booby, Juggler, Legerdemain,
Right Pages to bear up vain Glory's Train.
Can this be Honour to the *Britifh* Nation,
To gild her Book with Defamation?
As Slander harbours in the Dunghill Kind,
So Heroines abounds in a gen'rous Mind.
If Genealogy was underftood,
It's all a Farce, her Title is not good;
Can Seed of noble Blood, or renown'd 'Squires,
Teach Drudges to clean Spits, and build up Fires?
Two Preface Cullifs's goes far to fhow,
Whether the Pedigree be high or low;
Such Laws, Thrift, and meer Oftentation,
Sets forth th' great Roaft-ruler of the Nation.
Well has fhe marketed her little Wit,
By a great Artifice link'd clofe to it:

Poor

[v]

Poor cunning Art fometimes finds Ways to rife
Up to fuch Heights as might the World furprize;
Can Cream be thought a proper Sauce for Fifh,
Or Salmon bak'd in Milk a wholefome Difh?
If Epicures full of fuch Meat fhould cram,
Their Stomachs they might lofe, and the Cooks
    damn.
When Appetite is gone Health may depart,
But fhe relieves this by her Cook'ry Art:
A Chapter for the Sick fhe has prepar'd,
Wherein fhe fhews her Skill and great Regard;
Says, fhe meddles not in the Phyfick Way,
But Nurfe and Cooks muft her Precepts obey:
Directions proper for fick Ladies Meat,
Befides what Doctors fhall prefcribe to eat;
Her firft Charge given to Nurfe and Cook for
    Food,
Is Mutton and Roots be they bad or good,
To abate the Sicknefs or inflame the Blood.
Of Butchers Meat-gravy as ftrong as Glue,
To reftore Health and give them Spirits new;
And when fo weak as to take little Food,
Affirms the Cordial will do them moft Good:
To very weak Beef-broths a hearty Drink,
Let fainting Ladies on their Matron think;
Another Cordial Draught fhe has in Store,
And bids the Nurfe give the Sick one Draught
    more:

A

A Jill of Pork-broth in the Morning foon,
If their Stomachs will take the fame at Noon:
If Nurfe and Cook obey their Teacher's Will,
Sore may the Sick mourn at her uncouth Skill.
Bad does fhe boil, and full as ill fhe roafts,
Good Meat does fpoil, yet of her Cook'ry boafts.
Had fhe of *Tom Thumb* made a new Tranflation,
Such Dictates might divert the whole Nation:
So great a Progeny of Lady Blunder,
Might make Beaus laugh till their Sides burft
      afunder;
So many Criticks in Novel and Hift'ry,
Yet very few knows ought of the Cook's Myft'ry.
She muft defcend down from the Sapfcul Race,
That fuch great Surfeits gives fo bold a Grace;
And one likewife whofe Fancies was fcant,
Makes up a Book for to relieve that Want.
Here, there, and yonder Cook'ry Fragments ga-
      thers,
And dreffes up her Daw in borrow'd Feathers:
Adds to her Pickings up a Cook'ry Guefs,
Commits the grand Affair into the Prefs:
Cries, of all Books yet printed her's th' beft,
Read it but Maids, and foon your Dinner's drefs'd;
Be Kitchen Buftlers, learn both Trade and Trick,
Your Teacher fhews to furfeit whole and fick.
Then cries, who prints her Book or any Part,
She'll profecute for ftealing Cook'ry Art:

Look

[vii]

Look at the Lady in her Title Page,
How faft it fells the Book, and gulls the Age.
A Kitchen Dairy is the Lady's Book,
And fays, there's all Things fitting for the Cook.
Bids other Ladies fit and take their Eafe,
She'll teach them Cooks that fhall with Judgment
    pleafe:
Ignorant Maids fays, as they are great Sinners,
They'll buy the Book, and drefs up Ladies Din-
    ners:
And fpell and put together, it will read,
And in the Art of Cook'ry fhall proceed.
Famous Artift, great Kitchen Director,
Why might fhe not as well turn'd Architector?
Laid Plans for Houfes, fet forth Rules and Lines,
And bid the Ploughman build up her Defigns.
Delude illit'rate Men as well as Maids,
To profefs'd Builders and Mafters of Trades;
And when fhe's fill'd the World brim full of
    Wonder,
To fee her various Ways found out to plunder,
Vain Glory bratling forth like Blafts o'Thunder.
Sole Houfe Director of the *Britifh* Ifle,
Sounds out the Trumpet of Self-praifes, while
A profefs'd Cook, born in a homely Cottage,
Beholds the Surfeits of her Meat and Pottage;
Mufes upon the Purport of the Book,
With God fends Meat, but who could fend the
    Cook.

This

This Cottager efteems herfelf free-born,
That trick and bite, and all Impoftors fcorn.
She ne'er beheld the Splendour of a Court,
Nor has fhe Learning Rhetorick to fupport;
Had fhe known Grammar, might made better
    Rhyme,
Words more conneft, and of a Style fublime.
Criticks may pick the Faults out of her Satyr,
And fee the Want of Letters, not of Nature;
Or fay, the Lady might expeft Submiffion,
From one fo far beneath her in Condition.
To better Birth, fuperior Worth and Merit,
She Homage pays with Body, Soul, and Spirit;
Yet Criticizers Sentiments may pafs,
What Title can be due to broken Glafs:
But if th' Book want Juftice, Truth, and Reafon,
Fair regulating can't be deem'd a Treafon.
Cooks of found Judgment may be call'd difcreet,
Who ufe Precaution what they give to eat:
Would rather to their Breafts prefent a Knife,
As make known Surfeits to give Pain to Life.
Right Kitchen Cook'ry purifies the Blood,
Helps to keep Health and Conftitution good;
Which to preferve requires th' pureft Reafon,
Who corrupts Meat with Mixtures out o' Seafon,
Health impairs, and guilty is of Treafon:
Or teaches what they do not underftand,
Grudge not them getting publick Reprimand;

Or

Or claims an Art of which they are no Judge,
If they're detected by a labour'ng Drudge.
Who thinks the Crime on Artifice to foar,
The fame to lafh Impoftors till they roar:
She on a Proverb oftentimes have thought,
It's beft for Ladies what is deareft bought.
If fo her Cook'ry does them good,
Which to refine fhe many a hot Fire ftood;
Bought it with Health, Strength, and Refolution,
And paid for it a robuft Conftitution.
A Gem that far exceeds Talents of Gold,
For this fuperior Gem fhe fairly fold;
Oppref's'd with Akes and Pains, 'twas her Pleafure,
What gave thefe Pains brought forth th' Cook'ry
    Treafure.
In Perfecution her Soul did afpire,
To a Reward for what fhe loft by Fire;
Yet as the Drudge ne'er had a fervile Spir't,
Nothing fhe asks but what's due to Merit.
She want's no Praife, if fhe's not beft deferving,
In her flow Pace can keep herfelf from ftarving;
If Approbation is giv'n to her Myft'ry,
And fhe enabl'd to write out her Hift'ry:
The World will then fee which Way, what Way
    how
Hardfhips was laid for her to wreftle through;
Eighteen Years Cook, and Miftrefs of an Inn,
During the Whole encourag'd not lude Sin;
                   Dukes,

Dukes, Lords, Ladies, many worthy Esquire,
Came to her Inn, and often did admire,
How she found Cook'ry to fit all their Palates,
Both Nobles, Gentles, to de Chamber Valets:
T' please her virtuous Guests took great Delight,
Would not connive with Vice to gain their Mite.

A N

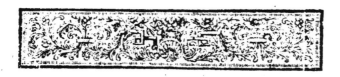

AN
ESSAY
ON THE
LADY's ART of COOKERY.

PLAIN Roafting and Boiling is a material Part of the Houfewife, when it is done to Perfection; and this is roafting and boiling to Perfection, when every feparate Order is punctually obeyed: Some love Mutton or Beef boiled very rear; fome love it thoroughly roafted or boiled; but at the fame Time to be fent up full of Gravy; others choofe it roafted or boiled to Rags: And every Mafter or Miftrefs expects their Roaft done to their Liking; and more or lefs roafted, requires more or lefs Time in roafting. All roaft Meat requires a clear brisk Fire; to be fpitted level, fo that the Fire plays equally round the Meat. I never falt Beef till it is fpitted, laid to the Fire, and bafted; then carefully ftrew Salt all over it, and it takes in as much as it requires. I never paper any Sort of Roafts for this Reafon, the Paper is a Hindrance to the Roafting, which waftes Time and Fire; and the Pins that holds it faft to the Roaft, are as many Taps after the Paper is taken off, that all the Gravy of the Meat runs out at: And here the Lady Teacher differs from me in her Charge to be fure to paper the Beef, and to bafte it all the Time it is roafting: This is a hard Task to the Cook, if fhe obeys her Teacher's Order, fhe will be half roafted herfelf if it is a large Piece of Beef; and if fhe baftes

A   it it all the Time it roafts with the hot Drippings, it will burn the Beef on the Outfide before it is thoroughly roafted. The Lady fays, that the Loins and Necks of Mutton are to be papered, and the Fat of the Loin of Veal; and if the Fat of the Loin of Veal be papered, what will become of the Lean of the Back of the Loin? It muft be burnt before the Kidney and Fillet be thoroughly roafted when it is papered: Therefore I advife none to paper the Fat of a Loin of Veal at any Rate; the bafting with Butter at laying down, and before it is drawn is right, but no papering. The Lady bids cut the Skin of a Loin of Pork a-crofs with a fharp Pen-knife, but forbids cutting the Skin of the Chine: But my Advice to all my Readers, is to make checker Work of the Chine as well as the Loin of Pork, left the Carver of it complain of the Cook. This Lady adds, that the beft Way to roaft a Leg, is firft to parboil it; this I call a Leg of Pork perfecuted: My Way of a roafted Leg of Pork, is to falt it with common Salt and Salt-petre, and let it lie a Week in a Tray, turning it three Times; then to fpit it and lay it down to the Fire, and put a Bottle of rough Cider into a very clean Dripping-pan, and bafte it with this all the Time it is roafting; and when it is enough, draw it on the Difh in which you fend it to the Table, take off the Skin; for Sauce, have fome boiled Apples and Sugar, and warm Vinegar and Muftard in the Difh: By this Way of roafting a Leg of Pork, it eats as delicious cold as hot; but half boiling the Leg, and then roafting, muft make a fad Martyr of that venerable Part of the Swine.

To roaft a Pig. Always contrive to lay the Pig down warm to the Fire that is newly killed and dreffed; put Sage cut fmall into the Belly of it, with a Cruft of Bread; then few up the Vent, fpit it, lay it down to the Fire and finge all the Hairs; then drudge it with Flour, and fo let it roaft till it is of

a

a light Brown; then take a Bunch of clean Feathers and whisk all the Flour clean from it; then take a little clean Beef or Mutton Drippings into a long Brafs-fpoon, and fet it into the Dripping-pan till it is melted, into which dip the Ends of the Bunch, whisk it with the Feathers, and when it is well greafed, throw all over it a handful of Salt; let the Fire be brisk all the Time it roafts; and when it is a dark Brown, duft off all the Salt with the Feathers, draw it before it lofe any of the Gravy. This Lady Teacher bids, duft it all over with Flour, and keep Flouring it all the Time it is roafting; this waftes Abundance of Flour and Time, and hinders the Pig from roafting. She adds, as foon as the Gravy begins to run from it, the Fire is to be ftirred up, Bafons to be fet into the Dripping-pan to receive the Gravy; Now every Bafon will take Tribute of the Gravy, and there is no Gravy fo preferable to its own mixed with melted Butter and the Brains, with a little of the Sage that is in the Belly of it. The illiterate Maid is by her Teacher's Order, to put a Quarter of a Pound of Butter into a coarfe Cloth, to rub the Pig after its Eyes have dropt out and Gravy run from it. Now in my Opinion this Pig muft be over-roafted before this Operation is perform'd, and if the Maid rub it with this coarfe Cloth till all the Butter is confumed, what Pig that ever was roafted could have a Skin to endure fuch a rubbing Bout? For by my Computation it would be a full half Hour, before fuch a Quantity of Butter could be confumed, as is in the coarfe Cloth; which would not only rub off all the young Animal's Skin of its Back, but the unskilled Hand rubbing muft make Execution into the Flefh; fo the martyr'd Pig fhews this roaft-ing to Perfection.

To roaft a Hare. If the Skin can be taken off clean, that there is none of the Down matted in the Flefh of the Hare; do not wafh her, but keep her Blood

with-

within her; make a Pudding of her Liver, Beef-suet, Thyme, Sweet-marjoram, Parſley, Shalot, an Egg, a little grated Bread, an Anchove cut ſmall; mix all together with Pepper, Nutmeg, and Salt, and put into the Belly of the Hare, and ſew it up; cut ſome Raſhers of Bacon, and with very ſmall wooden Skewers, prick theſe Raſhers on the Back and Buttocks of her; baſte her with Butter, and when ſhe is enough, have plain melted Butter in the Diſh, which the Company mixes with the ſavoury Pudding. The Lady Teacher has preſcrib'd for a large Hare, two Quarts of Milk and half a Pound of But-ter, which the Hare is to ſoak all up, and then ſhe will be enough, and to have a fit Sauce: A Pint of Cream, and half a Pound of Butter muſt, in my Opi-nion, take all the Taſte of the Hare from her, and ſhe muſt be a boil'd Hare, for I cannot think her roaſted; nor can ſhe be palatable, nor ſo much Cream to ſo little Fleſh wholeſome, but pernicious to Health.

To roaſt Veniſon. A large Hanch of Veniſon, make Paſte, and roll as thin as a Lid for a Family ſtanding Pye; lay this all over the Veniſon, but put no Butter in the Paſte; lay whitiſh brown Paper all over the Paſte, and roaſt it at a briſk Fire: A large Hanch will take ſix Hours roaſting, the Paſte keeps the Fat of the Veniſon from waſting; have boil'd Bread, Water, and Cinnamon, put Half the Quantity of Red-wine, and ſweeten it with Sugar; ſend up the Sauce in a Sauce-baſon; the Veniſon will have Gra-vy ſufficient for the Diſh.

To roaſt Ducks. Be ſure to pick the Ducks well, be cautious in drawing the Guts, cut not to burſt them, lay them warm to the Fire with Sage and Onion within them; the Necks, Livers, and Gizzards boil'd with a little Onion and Pepper will be Gravy, and Red-wine Sauce for them.

To roaſt Pigeons. By no Means roaſt them on the poor Man's Spit with the ſix Hooks at the End, for
this

this Reason; the Backs of the Pigeons will be raw
when their Breasts are roasted, then they are all to be
turn'd their Backs to the Fire; besides the Danger
of dashing the Pigeons against the Barrs, by the
Swinging of the String; as they must be untracta-
ble Rope-dancers: Lay them warm to the Fire with
Parsley and Butter in their Bellies; let them have a
clear Fire, and the long Spit against the Beggar's
Spit, most Gravy for any Money; let the Sauce be
Parsley and melted Butter. In the Chapter of *Roasts*
and *Boils*, the Lady Teacher has recommended the
Twining-band as the best Way to roast a Pigeon;
and in her second Chapter of *Made Dishes*, is the
Piece of Iron with six Hooks at the End, on which
the Pigeons are to be roasted: And where she, this
Teacher says, the Pigeons will swim with their own
Gravy, although Reason told me the Contrary; yet
I was Fool enough to believe that there might be
some Magick Art in the long String tyed to the
Chimney Top, by which Art the Pigeons might receive so much more Gravy than any other Pigeons ever
known to have; so I fulfilled the Order, for I filled
the Pigeon full of Butter and Parsley, tyed the String
(according to Order) to the Chimney, and when I
had perform'd all this Operation with a Pigeon, I
found less Gravy in it than there would have been if
it had been roasted in the common Way; besides
this single Pigeon had double the Advantage of the
Six, as it had all the Fire playing round it as it was
turning, which Part I very diligently perform'd, as
at that Time I had a proper Kitchen, which was my
Bed-chamber, whose Chimney-piece was very suitable
for a poor Man's Spit: Now as one Pigeon was so
far from answering such a Quantity of Gravy, as to
make it swim, how much worse will the Six hang
on six Hooks, for the Fire can but play half Round
them, for their Breasts must screen their Backs, or
their Backs must screen their Breasts, so that by turning

ing them muſt conſume their Juice; but if the Pigeon be done by the skillfulleſt Cook in the Univerſe, ſtill it is but a Pigeon, and cannot diſcharge Gravy to make it ſwim in the Diſh; but the poor Man's Spit is a Deſtroyer of the Gravy, and not a Preſerver of it. And as to Fowls roaſting, to tell to a Minute the Time they take roaſting, there ſhould be an exact Diſtance from the Fire, for the Illiterate and Ignorant may very eaſily err in proportioning the proper Diſtance of the Spit from the Fire; and in Caſe you be ſo fortunate as to find it out, you may do very well in roaſting a large Turkey and a ſmall one. Likewiſe in roaſting a Gooſe, the ſame may be obſerved; but if it is a clear Fire and at a proper Diſtance from it, the Gooſe will loſe her Gravy; for an Hour will roaſt the beſt Gooſe I ever ſaw. By her Rules for Roaſting, there is an Hour and a Quarter, and no Fowl is ſo inſipid as a Gooſe ſerv'd up without her Gravy. I had a very worthy Gueſt that did practice the Law, was a Critick in no Part of Cookery but in a Gooſe roaſting, and he would ſee the Fire and the Gooſe laid down, and never allowed more then Forty-five Minutes; he had his Watch by him, and would not let the Gooſe have one Minute more than the above forty-five Minutes; then there was a Diſh full of the Gravy of the Gooſe. By theſe Rules a wild Duck is to have ten Minutes roaſting, Woodcocks, Snipes, and Partridges, will take Twenty. Now ſuppoſe there is Woodcocks and wild Ducks for Dinner, the Ignorant and Illiterate are by theſe Rules of their Teacher, to lay the Woodcocks to the Fire five or ten Minutes before the Ducks; and if the Ducks are well roaſted, the Woodcocks muſt certainly be over-much; for a Woodcock will but take half the Time of a wild Duck's roaſting.

As to Roots and Greens boiling. Why a wooden Veſſel is not proper to waſh or lay the Greens in, for Duſt and Dirt may hang round a Pan as well as

a

a Pail, and a Pail is more common to wash or lay Greens in for Kitchen Use, and may be sooner cleaned than a Pan. No Meat is to be boiled with the Greens, for that discolours; but I rather think that the Greens would discolour the Meat. Use no Iron Pan to them, for they are not proper, but let them be Copper, Brass, or Silver. I think I durst venture a Wager, to boil Greens in an Iron Pan, as well as this Lady-Teacher shall boil in a Silver one. All Sorts of young Sprouts is by this Teacher's Order to be boiled in a great deal of Water, and when the Stalks falls to the Bottom they are enough. I differ from the Teacher in boiling young Sprouts in a great deal of Water; old Sprouts or Winter Cabbage will take a great deal of boiling; but young Sprouts the less Water, and the closer they are boiled, the brighter Green they will be: But if young Sprouts are put into a great deal of Water, and boiled till the Stalks fall to the Bottom, the Sprouts will be boiled very Yellow; which will make a very bad Appearance amongst a Company of Gentlemen and Ladies at a Table.

In Parsnips boiling. They require a great deal of boiling, and you may know when they are soft by running a Fork into them; a Fork may get entrance into a Parsnip before it is boiled at all, although it will not enter so easily as when it is boiled soft, which you may know as well by your Finger and Thumb pressing it, and the Fork may not be so ready; after they are boiled they are to be taken up and all the Dirt to be carefully scraped off them: But I advise you to scrape all the Dirt off them before they are put into the Pot to boil, were it but for the Sake of your Hands; for you will find it much easier scraping a cold Parsnip than a boiling hot one; besides it is more like a good Housewife to wash and scrape the Dirt off them before they are boiled.

The

The Boiling a Collyflower. Is ordered by this Teacher to be cut in four and boiled in a Sauce-pan; then taken up, and one half stewed in a Hash-pan, in a Pan full of Water, a Dust of Flour, and a Quarter of a Pound of Butter: But my Advice is to boil the Collyflower in clean Water; make Sauce of the Quarter of the Pound of Butter; and send up the Collyflower in a Dish, and the Butter in a Sauce-bason, for this Reason: The ten Minutes which is ordered to stew the one half of the Flower, will perhaps starve the other half; this is saving Trouble and likewise Butter; for if the Flower be turned and shaked according to her Order, the stewed will take up all the Butter; and there must be more Butter drawn for the boiled half of the Collyflower, as the Hash-pan will take Tribute of the Butter.

In dressing Artichokes. You are ordered to wring off the Stalks, and put them in cold Water with the Tops down, that all the Dust and Sand may boil out, and an Hour and a half will boil them: But my Advice is to cut the Stalks from them, and wash off all the Dust and Sand before they are put into the Pot, and not to trust to the Water boiling the Sand and Dust out of them; for instead of boiling out the Sand and Dust, and Twitchbells, which are often lodged there, the boiling may obstruct the Passage, and I am apt to think that it would rather boil them further into the Artichoke: If this Advice be reasonable, take it, if not, thy Will be done. But it is amazing to me, that the Lady should order burnt Butter, for thickening Sauces, or to boil Butter in a Pan till it is Brown, and stir Flour into it till it is thick, and to put it by and keep it for Use: She likewise makes Use of this for thickening and browning Sauces; and adds, that there are few Stomachs that they agree with, therefore it is seldom to be used: But my Advice to you is, never to use it at all, don't give thy Master or Lady a known Offender to the Stomach;

mach; for in fo doing you deftroy their Appetite
and impair their Health; and confider what a Risk
you run in giving Offence to great Ones, notwithftanding you have got your Teacher's Commiffion to
ufe it feldom: 'Tis as much as to fay, that if the Family pleafes me, they fhall not have burnt Sauces;
but if they vex or difoblige me, they fhall meet with
a burnt Butter Stomach Tincture; which by ftanding
a little Time, will be as ftrong as Whale Oil: So
has this Lady Inftructor taught her Pupils, to revenge themfelves on their Superiors if offended.

In Page 24, is a white Fricaffey. To boil three
Chickens tender in Milk and Water; and to throw
away what they were boiled in. But my Advice is
to let alone the Milk, and carefully preferve the
Chicken Broth, it being a Cordial to a tender Stomach, or is a help to rich Broths; but throwing
the Broth away, is doing an Injury to your Mafter
and Miftrefs. And although fome are of Opinion that
Milk and Water boil the Chickens white, I aver
the Contrary; Milk will curdle, and boil them blacker
than Water alone. I have feen great want of one
fingle Chicken for the Sake of the Broth, and could
not be had for Love or Price: And does this anfwer
the thrifty Lady Teacher's Propofals and Pretences?

In Page 29, Is a Breaft of Veal in Hodge-podge. Cut
your Breaft of Veal into fmall Pieces, and fry it brown
with Half a Pound of Butter put into a Stew-pan;
and fill'd up with Water, green Peafe, hot Spices,
fweet Herbs, Lettice, and Onions; if no Peafe, three
or four Cucumbers, Sellery; and if no Lettice, Cabbage Sprouts: And if you would have a very fine
Difh, fill your Lettice with Force-meat, and tie the
Tops clofe with Thread: Place your Lettice in the
Middle, and the Meat all round it; then pour on
your Sauce. Thus the Lady orders her delicate Difh,
and fays, it will ferve Abundance of People: And I
believe it will, and have plenty of Fragments remaining.

ing. The Lady is a little out of her Element touching her Lettice binding; for before the Meat can be done, the Bindings of her Lettice will be unloosed, in spight of all her profound Wisdom in Cookery.

In Page 31st, *Is to Collar a Breast of Mutton.* Do it the same Way, and take off the Skin; and it eats very well, says the Lady.

And likewise prescribes another Way of cooking Mutton, by collaring it as above, and basting it with Half a Pint of Wine; and when it has drunk the Wine well up, baste it with Butter and Gravy. But in my Opinion, the Mutton will be so strongly intoxicated with the Wine, that it will be apt to lothe the Butter and Gravy.

And the Lady further adds, that the Inside of a Sirloin of Beef is very good done the above Way; and if you don't approve of Wine, a Quart of Milk, and a Quarter of a Pound of Butter, to baste the Inside of your Sirloin. Here I disagree with the celebrated Instructor; and advise you not to fuddle the Mutton with Wine; nor take out the Inside of the Sirloin of Beef, which is the most juicy Part of it; nor surfeit it with Milk; nor spoil a good roasting Piece of Beef, by robbing it of it's most delicious Part.

In Page 34, *To force the Inside of a Sirloin of Beef.* She orders to take out all the Flesh to the Bone. But I advise you by no Means to take it from the Bone; because, after thou hast taken the Flesh, and made Force-meat with Suet and Bread, How then wilt thou get this fine Meat to stick to the Bone again? A Fillet of Beef, of a Steer, or spav'd Quay, or a thorough fed Cow, will weigh eight or nine Pounds; besides the Suet, Bread, and other Ingredients, thus laid on the Bone again; the Fat skewer'd down upon it, and over that a Paper; yet notwithstanding, the Force-meat will make Way through Fat and Paper into the Dripping-pan: Although the
Teacher's

Teacher's Order is not to let the Paper be taken off till the Meat is in the Dish; yet the Fat and Paper will not have Strength to bear up the Force-meat; so that fall it must, if it be done as this Teacher orders. There is much Labour lost, and the Sirloin is disfigured; besides the Fillet would have been better plain roasted; than by all this stupid, expensive Art of the Lady Teacher's.

I come now to shew the Extravagancy of the rolled Rump of Beef. For there is the Flesh of two Fowls, Beef-suet, cold Ham, and Abundance of other Items: But you will gain more Credit by keeping the Rump whole, and save your Master's Charges. For by *P.* 35. The rolled Beef is to boil eight or ten Hours in a Pot that can just hold it; and yet this Pot is to be fill'd with Water: But as the Bones are taken out of it, it will pack so close in the Pot, as to leave Room for very little Water; so that Reason would dictate, that eight or ten Hours is sufficient to boil the Pot dry. But the Teacher thinks that the Sauce will not be boil'd enough, as she, has ordered the Beef to be taken up till it is better boil'd: And to add red Wine, Yolks of Eggs, Butter and Flour; and when it is enough, to pour it over the Meat. Though many Rumps, Sirloins, and Beef Buttocks are destroyed; yet it's much if you keep the Pot-bottom from burning.

In Page 37. The Lady's Beef Collops are made thus: They are to be ten Minutes in scalding Water, with sweet Herbs; and sent to Table.

Next are *stew'd Beef-stakes.* First, stew the Stakes in Water, Wine, Butter, Flour, and Herbs; then to flour and fry them.

To Fry Beef-stakes. Take Half a Pint of Ale that is not bitter; and fry them in Rump-stakes.

Her second Way is to fry them in Butter, as much as will grease the Pan; to cut off the Fat, and fry it by itself, and the Lean by itself.

Ano-

Another Way to do Beef-ftakes: Is to half broil them; then put them in a Stew-pan with Pepper, Salt, Gravy, and Butter rolled in Flour; and let them ftew Half an Hour. But her rolled beef-ftakes exceed; for four Beef-ftakes there are to be Force-meat made of the Flefh of a large Fowl, a Pound of Veal, Half a Pound of cold Ham, the Kidney-fat of a Loin of Veal, Sweet-bread cut in Pieces, the Yolks of four Eggs, an Ounce of Truffles, Morels, Pepper, Salt, and half a Pint of Cream; thefe fhe pounds all together, and lays upon the Stakes: Which in my Opinion, will be about ten Pounds of Force-meat, to her four Beef-ftakes; and is a fufficient Quantity of Force-meat for twenty Difhes.

The Kidney-fat of a good Loin of Veal, by my Computation, muft weigh three Pounds; the Flefh of a large Fowl, (I call a Turkey) three Pounds; a Pound of Beef-fuet; Veal Sweet-bread, Half a Pound; a Pound of Veal; and Half a Pound of Ham; Eggs, Cream, Truffles, Morels, Herbs, and Seafoning, I call a Pound; this makes up the above Computation: Of which I propofe to make five very good Difhes; Three of which Subftantial, with the Help of a Pound of Spice, and a Pound of Flour: There can be no lefs than a Pound and a Half of Beef, to roll two Pounds and a Half of Force-meat in each Stake; for the four Stakes I have fix Pounds of Beef, of which I make a very good Ragoo; the Kidney Fat of the Loin of Veal, will make Stuffing for the Turkey's Crop, and Force-meat to the other Difhes; the Pound of Veal, and half Pound of Bacon, with the Help of the Force-meat, will make a Side-difh of Scotch Collops; the Sweet-bread, with Half an Ounce of the Truffles and Morels, will make a Fricaffey; the Pound of Beef-fuet, Cream, and the Eggs, with the Pound of Flour, and a Pound of Fruit, will make a Hunter's Pudding; the other half Ounce of Truffles and Morels, with Force-meat Balls,

Balls, Mushrooms, and the Gravy, that the Lady
orders to the Beef-stakes, I thus divide; three half
Jills of it I give to the Ragoo; the other half Jill to
the Scotch Collops; and white Sauce to the Fricassey: So I set my Ragoo at the Head; my roast Turkey at the Foot; the Hunter's Pudding in the Middle;
one Side is the Collops; the Fricassey the other: All
these cram'd together would be a Surfeit; separate
them in the above Manner, and they may appear before a Nobleman.

Reason is a notable Instructor in Cookery; it
teaches the profess'd Cook to have Mercy on the
Master's Property, and not wilfully to destroy his
Substance, by making such Havock, as Beef-stakes
have done in all the Shapes now mentioned; for
none of them are fit to appear at the Table of a Gentleman: And to see the Beef defac'd, and so shame-
fully wasted, would be a great Crime in any Person
not to detect.

In Page 43, Is to roast Ox Palates. To boil them
tender, and cut them in Slices two Inches long; to
lard Half with Bacon; to have three Pigeons; three
Chicken Peepers, to be filled with Force-meat, and
nicely larded; to spit them thus, a Bird, a Sage-leaf,
and a Piece of Bacon, till all is spited.

To lard Cocks-combs. Parboil Oysters, and Lamb-
stones with Bacon; spit and roast them with Sage-
leaf and Bacon between them; baste them with
Bread grated, the Yolks of Eggs, and Nutmeg, all
the Time they are roasting. Now the Query is, how
these tender Lamb-stones and Cocks-combs, but more
especially the larded Oysters, will endure the Buffets
of the Bread and Eggs? the Oysters will baste to
pieces, and beyond Art to keep them on the Spit;
although the Task will be hard to lard a parboil'd
Oyster; yet if large it may be done: But where to
find a Stomach to digest these larded Oysters with
Bacon, will be the greatest Hardship.

In

In Page 50, *To bake Lamb and Rice.* Take a
Neck and Loin of Lamb, and half roaſt it; boil
half a Pound of Rice in a Quart of Gravy, till it is
thick; and ſtir in a Pound of Butter the Yolks of
ſix Eggs; butter the Diſh all over; dip the Stakes
into melted Butter; lay them in the Diſh, and pour
three Yolks of Eggs over the Rice; bake it in an
Oven half an Hour. The half Pound of Rice is butter'd extravagantly; boiled in Gravy, it ſeems to be
a Pudding: But a Gravy Rice Pudding is as uncom-
mon as it ſeems to be unreaſonable; for the Pound of
Butter being ſtirred into the Rice; the Diſh butter'd
over; the Stakes dipt in melted Butter, will take
another Pound, and muſt make a great Well of Oil
upon the Rice and Lamb: For it will be far out of
the Power of the Rice to keep them from ſwim-
ming. To me it ſeems to be a Surfeit to a hungry
Plough-man.

In Page 52, *To ſtew a Lamb or Calf's Head.* She
takes for Force-meat two Pounds of Veal, and two
Pounds of Beef-ſuet, to be chopt all together; two
ſtale Rolls to be grated, four Yolks of Eggs, two
Anchovies, with other Seaſoning. But my Advice
is, never to make half a Pound of Force-meat for a
Calf's Head; and Half that Quantity for a Lamb's,
is ſufficient: Although this Lady Teacher has between five or ſix Pounds of Force-meat; beſides a
Jill of Oyſters, Muſhrooms half a Pint, Truffles,
Morels, and more Muſhrooms; it is very great Extravagancy.

In Page 54, *Is bombarded Veal.* Out of a Fillet
of Veal, cut five lean Pieces as thick as your Hand;
to which is ordered five Sheep Tongues to be larded; then make a well ſeaſoned Force-meat of Veal,
Bacon, Ham, Anchovy. And to make another tender Force-meat of Veal, Beef-ſuet, Muſhrooms,
Spinage, Parſley, Thyme, Sweeet-marjoram, Winter-
ſavoury, green Onions, Pepper, and Mace: The well
ſeaſoned

seasoned is to be baked for the Middle; the other is to be fill'd by Way of *Bolognia* Sausage; to boil it, and then cut and fry it: So there is Force-meat baked, boiled, and fry'd. Thus by Mismanagement, the Vulgar in this Country often are Sufferers: For when their Market is made, they will have roasted, boiled, and baked; but in the latter End of the Week they suffer Hunger. And indeed I cannot help comparing the Lady's bombarded Veal to vulgar Extravagancy.

Scotch Collops *à la Francois*. Cut a Leg of Veal into very thin Collops, and lard them with Bacon, and pour boiling Ale over them, to take out the Blood; to pour the Ale off into a Bason; to fry the Veal in Butter; the Collops laid in a Dish with toasted Bacon round it; the Ale to be put in a Stew-pan, with a Glass of Wine, Nutmeg, Pepper, two Anchovies, and a Piece of Butter: This is monstrous Sauce, for there is neither Gravy nor Water in it; but Ale and Wine thickened with Yolks of Eggs, Butter and Anchovies.

In Page 56, *Are larded* Scotch Collops. A Fillet of Veal is to be cut into thin Slices; the Skin and Fat is to be cut off; lard them with Bacon; fry them Brown; pour out all the Butter; lay the Collops on a Dish; take a Quarter of a Pound of Butter, melt it in the Pan, and strew in a Handful of Flour; stew it till they be Brown; and put three Pints of Gravy, with Herbs and Onion; the Collops to be put in and stew'd Half a Quarter of an Hour; and the Yolks of two Eggs, Force-meat Balls, a Piece of Butter, some Mushrooms; stir all together a Minute or two till all is thick. Reason says, that the burnt Butter and a Handful of Flour might make the Gravy thick enough, without the Yolks of Eggs. When this Teacher bid put by the burnt Butter for Use; she did not tell what Quantity was to be put in to thicken and brown the Gravy for a Made-dish. But
if

if her Readers have Penetration, they may find out
the Quantity in Larded *Scotch Collops* : By which
Collops, the Gentry may see the Teacher's Care of
giving their Stomachs Offence.

In her *Calf Head Surprise*: The Teacher proposes
a Task, that she cannot perform herself, if she do it
as she has prescribed to others; which is to bone the
Head, and fill it with a Ragoo, as in the Form it
was before ; it is to be fill'd with Sweat-breads,
Cocks-combs, Truffles, Morels, Mushrooms, Artichoke-bottoms, Asparagus-tops, stew'd in Gravy seasoned, Cream, Yolks of Eggs, and White-wine added
to the Ragoo; to keep it stirring one Way for fear of
turning; making it thick and smooth with Butter and
Flour. This choice collected Ragoo, with twenty
Force-meat Balls, is to be put into the Head; and
then to be fastened with fine Skewers; Force-meat
laid over it; and the Yolks of Eggs, Pieces of Butter over all the Head; to be bak'd two Hours in an
Oven. Indeed my Opinion is, that this Calf's Head
Surprise very well brooks its Name; and plainly
makes manifest the Teacher's Art of Cookery: For
if she had but made a Trial, she would then have seen
into the Error of her Imagination; Can a reasonable
Person believe that this Ragoo could have the Strength
of the Bones of the Calf's Head, to bear it up in the
Form it was before the Bones was taken out? For if
she had the true Art of Cookery, she would not have
made this choice Collection of tender Rarities into a
Ragoo, ready for dishing up; thickening it with
Cream and Eggs; giving Orders to turn it one Way,
for fear of breaking; and after it is smooth and
thick, to put it into the raw Calf's Head, to bake two
Hours: During which Time, what must become of
the thick smooth Sauce? Would not the Yolks of
Eggs break it into Tears of Envy, for the Indignity
done the Ragoo? What was the Ornament of every
Dish, is now become Stuffing for a Calf's Head:
Which

Which inftead of raifing it into its Form, makes it
an Object of Infamy : The Force-meat all bedaub'd
and baked upon it, muft appear at the Table, as if
the Head was fcabbed : And the Rivers of Tears
from the Ragoo, difcharg'd out of the Eyes, Ears,
and Mouth, muft have the Symptoms of the Glan-
ders in the Head : But when it is cut up, what a
Hodge-podge will the baked Ragoo make in their
various Colours. A Gentleman Critick, when he
fees the fcabbed Head appear at the Table, would
fwear it had been feized with the Plague, by the
Botches, Biles, and Marks of Violence upon it.

In Page 59, A Ham à la Braife. Slices of Beef
and Bacon, Herbs and Roots, are laid in the Bottom
of a Kettle; upon which lies the Ham, with the fat
Side uppermoft; which is ordered to be covered
with Slices of Beef, Bacon, Herbs, and Roots; to
be covered clofe with a Lid, and pafted; Fire to be
put under and over it; to be ftewed twelve Hours
with a flow Fire. A Ham indeed may be *à la
Braifed*; but it will take a large Quantity of Slices
of Beef and Bacon to keep it gently boiling twelve
Hours in the Juice of this Beef and Bacon, as there
is no Water ordered : A middling Ham will weigh
fourteen Pounds; Beef and Bacon to difcharge as
much Juice as will ftew the Ham twelve Hours,
Fire under and over it : The leaft that I can compute is fix Stone of Beef and Bacon; and if there
is, after it has ftewed twelve Hours, a Pint of Gravy, it will be furprifing, when the Fat is skim'd off,
if the Fat and Gravy will part; as Ham-fat is more
clammy than any other Fat. The Teacher has recommended this Liquor to be Sauce for a Ragoo to
the Ham; which fhe fays will do as well as Effence
of Ham. It is a ftrange Effence; but the pernicious
Part of the Strength of the Ham is fo ftrong, that a
hungry Hound from the Field would refufe it : But
fince this is fo plain a Demonftration, Who could
believe

believe that a Lady would prescribe a Dish so extravagant, and likewise Sauce fit to surfeit a Sow?

The Excellency of the Teacher's Taste and Fancy is further set forth, by various Ways of dressing a Pig: The Pig is to be skin'd up to the Ears; and a good Plumb-pudding Batter to be made of Milk, Eggs, Flour, and Beef-fat; the Skin to be fill'd and baken in the Form of a Pig. But what would this Artist say, if the Eggs make the Pudding rise in the baking, and leap out of the Skin? had she not better have boil'd it in a Bag, than to have robbed it of its Skin, for a Bag for her Pudding. Although she has told how to dispose of the four Quarters, by roasting them with Well-cresses and Mint-sauce; or to fry them with Spinage; or Ragoo it, for a Top-dish, the first Course; or a Bottom-dish, the Second; or white Fricassey it for a Top, or Side-dish, the second Course: But after all, it would have been better roasted, with the favourite Piece, even the Skin beautifully crisped.—Next it is to be skin'd, and filled with Force-meat, made of two Pounds of young Pork fat and lean, two Pounds of Veal; the same to fill it, and sew it up; and either roast or bake it, after the Skin is taken off. Query, How will this Pig's Belly hold the four Pounds of Pudding? And will not its Weight give it a fall into the Dripping-pan? Or you may have a very good Pye of it; as you see in the *Chapter* for *Pyes*: Or you may spit, and let it roast till it is thoroughly warm; then cut it into twenty Pieces, and stew them in a Pint of White-wine, and a Pint of strong Broth: Or cut off the Head, and divide the Quarters, and lard them with Bacon, and lay a Leaf of fat Bacon at the Bottom of the Kettle; upon which lay the Pig's Head, and the four Quarters, Bay-leaves, Lemon, Currans, Parsnips, Parsley; and cover all with Bacon, stewed in strong Broth.

A

A Pig Matelote. The Pig to be quartered; to be put into a Stew-pan, upon Slices of Bacon; to be covered with more Slices of Bacon; to be stewed in a Bottle of Wine: And when it is half done, cut two large Eels in six Inches Lengths; stew them with a Dozen of boiled Craw-fish: Scum the Fat off the Liquor that they were stew'd in; add to it a Pint of strong Gravy, thickened with burnt Butter.

A Pig like a fat Lamb. The Pig is to be trussed up like a Lamb, when it is cut through the Middle, and skin'd, parboil it; then throw Parsley over it; roast and drudge it: Let your Sauce be half a Pound of Butter, and a Pint of Cream, stewed all together till it is smooth.

To roast a Pig with the Hair on. Cut off its Feet, and truss it, prick up the Belly, spit it; lay it to the Fire, but take Care not to scorch it; and when the Skin begins to rise up in Flisters, pull off the Skin and Hair; and also baste it with Butter and Cream; or half a Pound of Butter, and a Pint of Milk: Drudge it with Crumbs of Bread, till it is half an Inch thick: The Sauce is to be Gravy and Butter; or else half a Pound of Butter, and a Pint of Cream.

The Pig newly killed, to be roasted with the Skin on. A Hard-meat made of a Pint of Cream, Yolks of Eggs, grated Bread, and Beef-suet; with Seasoning made in a stiff Pudding; its Belly is to be stuffed; and then to be spitted and laid to the Fire: And drudge it with Flour and Lemon-peel, and a Pint of Red-wine in the Dripping-pan; and when it is enough, shake Flour over; and send it up with a fine Froth: The Sauce in the Dripping-pan is to be thickened with Butter: You are to take great Care no Ashes fall into the Dripping-pan; which may be prevented by making a good Fire, which will not want any stiring. In my Opinion, the Teaching Lady has tried all the Ways of dressing a Pig, but the right one, and that she has not touch-

ed

ed upon: And if her Stomach can digeſt ſuch Food, as ſhe preſcribes in her various Ways of dreſſing a Pig, it will be very hard to diſturb it: For the various Tortures ſhe puts the poor Pig to, might give juſt Suſpicion, that the Teacher's Deſire is to waſte and conſume Wealth by Extravagancy, and create good Buſineſs to the Doctor. How often is the Pig robb'd of its Skin, the moſt delicious Morſel, and liked by every Body: Can Cream and Butter be proper Sauce for the Pig, or Eels, Craw-fiſh, and ſo much Bacon to ſtew with it? Who would bid roaſt a Pig with the Hair on; and order both Skin and Hair to be torn off together, even when it is roaſting? Although it is rather more decent than to ſend it to the Table with the Hair on. But if I had ſeen the Operation made on it at the firſt, without reading the Orders, I would certainly have thought the Cook had broke out of *Bedlam:* For none in their Senſes could perform Cookery ſo inconſiſtent with Reaſon.

In Page 70, *To dreſs a Turkey or Fowl to Perfection.* Bone them, and make Force-meat of the Fleſh of a Fowl, a Pound of Veal, half a Pound of Beef-ſuet, as much Crumbs of Bread, Muſhrooms, Truffles and Morels cut ſmall, ſweet Herbs and Spices; all this is made into Force-meat, with Yolks of Eggs; and the Turkey to be filled with. If Extravagance will dreſs the Turkey to perfection, it is not wanting; but it is attended with great Hazard of being very imperfectly roaſted.

Then there is *To ſtew a Turkey brown the nice Way.* It is to be boned, and fill'd with Force-meat, made thus; the Fleſh of a Fowl, half a Pound of Veal, the Fleſh of two Pigeons, a well pickled or dry'd Tongue, peal and chop it all together, and beat it in a Morter with the Marrow of a Beef-bone, or a Pound of Kidney-fat of a Loin of Veal. I ſay, a Tongue is a good Diſh in any Town in *England:*

A

A pretty Side-difh may be made of a good Fowl:
Two Pigeons may make another by good Management: And the true Art of Cookery, this half
Pound of Veal, and the Pound of the Kidney-fat of
the Loin of Veal, may make another: But if you
chop all thefe together, it is but one; and in my O-
pinion, a very aukward one too. For, after all this
Stuffing is put into the Turkey, it's to be put into
a Pot that will juft hold it; fo that the Bones being
taken out of it, and fo much Force-meat ftuffed in,
and put into a Pot that juft holds it; and as there
is no Bones in it, it muft be in the Shape of the
Pot; becaufe the Pot will be a Mould to fhape it:
As an additional and needlefs Expence, is Mufhrooms, Truffles, Morels, and Oyfters ftewed, and
put into little Loafs to furround this Turkey. Now,
I think, I could make fix tolerable Difhes out of
this intolerable one: I would boil my well pickled Tongue with Turnips, for the Head: Make a
Side-difh of the Fowl: Paradife my Pigeons, for the
Middle: Of the half Pound of Veal, and the Pound
of Kidney-fat, I would make a Side-difh of Veal-
olives: My Oyfters, the other Side-difh: And I
would plain roaft my Turkey, for the Bottom.

To force a Fowl. The Teacher has a particular and
wonderful Method; the Skin is to be taken off the
Fowl firft, and then the Flefh pick'd from the
Bones, which is to be minced fmall; a Pound of
Beef-fuet fhred, and a Pint of large Oyfters chopt,
two Anchovies, a Shallot, grated Bread, and Sweet-
herbs fhred and mixed together, and wrought up
with Yolks of Eggs; all thefe are to be laid on the
Bones of the Fowl; the Skin to be drawn over all,
and fewed up the Back. The Teacher ought to
have ordered the Skin to be tann'd, to enable it to
ftand the Fire, and keep its Burden from falling into
the Dripping-pan, before it is half roafted: The
Teacher bids either boil it in a Bladder a Quarter of

an

an Hour, or roaſt it : But if is to be boil'd, is not a Pint of Oyſters ſufficient, without ſtewing. more which ſhe has ordered to be made for Sauce, for this Fowl? By which you may ſee the wild Extravagancy of her Cookery in every Article I mentioned. and all the Diſhes ſpoiled into the Bargain.

In Page 73, *Chicken Surpriſe.* Is as ſurpriſingly cook'd as any of the Reſt : The Chicken is to be roaſted ; for a ſmall Diſh one large Fowl ; the Lean to be taken from the Bone ; ſtew'd in ſeven Spoon-fuls of Cream, Butter and Flour ; then is ſeven Slices of Bacon to be cut, upon which is ſeven Rolls made of Force-meat, with a hollow Place in each Roll, into which is the ſtewed Chicken to be put ; cover-ed with Force-meat, and baked in an Oven ; the Rolls are to be the Height and Bigneſs of *French* Rolls : Each of which in my Opinion will take a Pound and a Half of Force-meat ; a ſufficient Quantity for twenty made Diſhes : And all this for the lean Fleſh of a Fowl to be baked in ; and recom-mended by the Teacher as a pretty Side-diſh for the firſt Courſe, Summer or Winter, when it can be got. I think you may have it all the Year round if you pleaſe, for Chickens or Fowls are never out of Seaſon both at once ; and it may be a large Top or Bottom-diſh : For ſeven Force-meat Rolls in the Size, as they are ordered, will fill a large Top-diſh with Gravy-ſauce ; and the Expence of as much Force-meat, may make four Top or Bottom-diſhes.

In Page 74, *Chickens roaſted with Force-meat and Cucumbers :* For two Chickens, take the Fleſh of a Fowl, and two Pigeons, and ſome Slices of Ham or Bacon, chop all well together ; ſoak the Crumb of a Penny Loaf in Milk, boil it, and when it is cool, mix all together ; and ſeaſon with Herbs and Spice. This is to ſtuff two Chickens ; and four Cucumbers, with the rich fry'd Gravy ſhe makes the Sauce, far exceed the Price of the Chickens.

Page 79th, Is to dress a Duck with Green Pease. A
deep Stew-pan to be put over the Fire, with fresh
Butter; into which is the Duck to be put, and turned two or three Minutes; then is the Fat to be put
out, and half a Pint of Gravy put to it; with two
Lettices cut small, a Bundle of Sweet-herbs, and a
Pint of Pease: Cover your Pan close, let them stew
half an Hour; then put Mace and Nutmeg; thick-
en it with Butter and Flour; or with the Yolks of
Eggs and Cream, three Spoonfuls.

Would not any reasonable Person think, that a
Pint of Green Peas and two Lettices, stewed half an
Hour in half a Pint of Gravy, would be thick e-
nough, if not over thick? I should think that it
would have rather wanted to be made thinner, than
to have Eggs and Cream to thicken it: For to me,
the Cream and Eggs would make a very odd Figure mixt with stew'd Lettices, Green Peas, and
a Duck.

In Page 83, Is a Goose à la Mode. Skin and bone
the Goose; take the Fat off it: Do a Fowl the
same Way; boil a dry'd Tongue; put the Fowl
and Tongue into the Goose; season all with Salt,
Pepper, and Mace; sew it up in the same Form it
was before, and put it into a little Pot that will just
hold it; put two Quarts of Beef-gravy to it, a Bundle of Sweet-herbs, an Onion, Slices of Ham, or
good Bacon, between it and the Fowl; let it stew
an Hour, and when it begins to boil take it up:
Add to the Gravy Red-wine, Sweet-bread of Veal,
Mushrooms, Butter, and Flour.

Now after all this Expence, the Goose is ill used,
so is the Tongue and Fowl; for it would have been
much better roasted with its Skin, Bones and Fat
on it; (I say this large fine Goose is very ill used)
for its own Gravy is sufficient for Sauce; with Apples boil'd, a little Vinegar, and Mustard, which
will not exceed Two-pence: The other Stuffing and
Sauce

Sauce will coſt ſix Shillings; yet at the ſame Time, the Teacher would have herſelf thought Thrifty, by adding *N. B.* To boil the Bones of the Gooſe and Fowl in the Gravy.

In Page 92, Is to dreſs Partridges à la Braiſe. Lard two Brace of Partridges with Bacon; grate Pepper, Salt, and Mace on them; lay in a few Slices of Bacon, Beef, and Veal in the Pan; upon which lay your Partridges, with Carrots, Onions, and Sweet-herbs; the Breaſts of them are to be downwards; Slices of Beef and Veal laid over them; ſtew them eight Minutes over a ſlow Fire, then give the Pan a ſhake, and put a Pint of boiling Water to them; ſtew them half an Hour, and then take up the Birds, and put in a Pint of thin Gravy, boil it to half a Pint; then take a Veals Sweet-bread, Truffles, Morels, Fowls-livers, and Cocks-combs, ſtew'd in a Pint of good Gravy half an Hour; adding Artichoke-bottoms, Aſparagus-tops, and Muſhrooms; add the other Gravy to this; put in your Partridges to heat; and if it is not thick enough, take Butter and Flour, toſs it up; or if you'll be at the Expence, take Veal, and Ham-cullis.

For Garniſhing two roaſted Partridges, and the Fleſh of a large Fowl, a little parboil'd Bacon, ſome Marrow or Beef-ſuet cut fine, Muſhrooms chopt ſmall, Truffles, Artichoke-bottoms, Mace, Pepper, Nutmeg, Salt, and Sweet-herbs chopt fine, the Crumb of a Two-penny Loaf ſoak'd in hot Gravy; mix all well together with the Yolks of two Eggs; make your Pains on Paper of a round Figure, and the Thickneſs of an Egg, form them with the Point of a Knife, which muſt be dipt in the Egg-yolk, in order to ſhape them; then neatly bake them a quarter of an Hour in a quick Oven.

Now, I think, I could make a Dinner for eight Gentlemen and Ladies, with the ſeparate Ingredients that are preſcrib'd to *Partridges à la Braiſe, Par-*

tridges Pains, to garnish, *&c.*——In the following Manner I make the Entertainment: With the Slices of Veal that are under and above the Partridges, I make a Dish of *Scotch* Collops with some of the Slices of Bacon that is under and over the Patridges, the Pint of thin Gravy, a little of the Seasoning, the Mushrooms that are first prescribed: And the Slices of Beef that are laid under and over them, I make a very good Beef-stake Pye; the Value of the overplus Bacon will make the Crust: The Fowls Livers and Cocks-combs will be a Fricassey, that may appear at a Prince's Table: A Veal's Sweet-bread, if it be a very good one, by the Help of Truffles, Morels, and half of the Pint of strong Gravy the other: The other Half of the Cocks-combs, and Fowls Livers, boil'd Asparagus, Toast and Butter, is a Side-dish: The Crumbs of a Two-penny Loaf will make a very good Pudding: The Gravy that it is soak'd in will make a very good Soop, by the Help of the Herbs and Roots that are ordered to the Partridges: A Ragoo of Artichokes is a pretty Dish: The large Fowl and Mushroom-sauce cannot be objected to for a Top-dish: And the Best of all is three Brace of Partridges, in their natural Shape and Taste, roasted with butter'd Crumbs.——So thus I place my Dinner: The large Fowl and Mushroom-sauce boil'd, at the Head; *Scotch* Collops at the Foot; the Soop in the Middle; one Side is a Fricassey of Fowls Livers, and Cocks-combs; Toasts and Asparagus the other: The second Course is my six roasted Partridges at the Top; Beef-stake Pye at the Bottom; Pudding in the Middle; one Side is the Sweet-bread; ragoo'd Artichokes the other; and has Gravy sufficient for all, besides the hot Gravy she orders the Bread to be soak'd in.—She adds, if you will be at the Expence, thicken it with Veal and Ham-cullis; but says she, it will be full as good without. In that I think her very right, for the Taste of the Partridges

D   were

were fo barbaroufly deftroyed before the Veal and Ham-cullis, which was no further required, than to add to the Surfeit, and enlarge the Expence.

In Page 93, *is a ftew'd Pheafant.* She bids the Pheafant be ftew'd in Veal Gravy, till there is e-nough for Sauce; and to parboil Artichoke-bottoms; and to roaft and blanch Chefnuts; and add to this Sauce, with Mace, Pepper, and White-wine, and fry'd Force-meat Balls.

Pheafant à la Braife. She bids lay a Lair of Beef all over your Pan, then a Lair of Veal, a Piece of Bacon, Carrot, Onion, fix Cloves of Mace, a Spoonful of Pepper, a Bundle of Sweet-herbs; then to lay in the Pheafant, then a Lair of Veal, and a Lair of Beef to cover it; then to fet it on the Fire fix Minutes, next to pour in two Quarts of boiling Water; let it ftew foftly an Hour and a Half; then orders to take up the Pheafant and keep it hot, and let the Gravy boil till there is about a Pint; then ftrain it off, and put it in again, and put in a Veal Sweet-bread, fome Truffles and Morels, fome Livers of Fowls, Artichoke-bottoms, Afparagus-tops, two Spoonfuls of Catchup, two of Red-wine, Butter, and Flour, fhake all together; put in your Pheafant, let them ftew all together, with a few Mufhrooms, about five or fix Minutes more; then take up your Pheafant, and pour your Ragoo all over with a few Force-meat Balls: You may lard it if you chufe.

Beautiful Bird how forry am I to fee thee fo tofs'd up with Inconfiftancies: I lived in a Family that took fuch Delight in their Pheafants, that neither Mafter nor Lady would fuffer the Game-keeper to fhoot any wild Fowl in the Wood, where the Pheafants inhabited, for fear of frightening them into the neighbouring Woods: That Gentleman had been at fome Expence in procuring a Brood of them, which he took fuch Care to preferve and increafe, that there was never one feen at his Table, although none in the North entertained more grandly then he did: He would let his Company see his fine Birds, but at the same Time said they must not taste them. He told a Nobleman, that these Birds had been very safely protected by him, for he had let them increase and multiply these nine Years, without taking one Bird out of their Flock: And as long, said he, as I'm Master of that Wood, none shall disturb them; they are my Harmony in the Summer Mornings and Evenings. Had he ordered a Pheasant to have been dressed, how far would he have been disappointed, had it been stewed with Chesnuts, and Artichoke-bottoms; or *à la Braised* with so many strong Mixtures, which would not leave the least natural Taste; beside the unnecessary Trouble and extravagant Expence. She says, for a roasted Pheasant, have Gravy in the Dish, and Bread-sauce in Plates; or scalded Well-cresses laid under it; or make Sellery-sauce stewed tender, strained and mixed with Cream, and poured into the Dish. She says, a *Frenchman* would order Fish-sauce to them, but then you'll quite spoil your Pheasants. But I say, that Sellery and Cream are not so proper Sauce as some Fish-sauce is: For many use plain Butter for Fish-sauce, which would be more proper Sauce than Sellery, Cream, and scalded Well-cresses to surfeit Pheasants. Her Fancy extends itself to great Lengths in wild Fowl spoiling.

In Page 95, Snipes in a Sourtout, or Woodcocks. Take Force-meat, made with Veal, Beef-suet, an equal Quantity of Crumbs of Bread, Mace, Pepper, Salt, Parsley, and Sweet-herbs; mix them with the Yolk of an Egg; lay some of this Meat round the Dish; then lay in the Snipes, being first drawn and half roasted: Take Care of the Trail, chop it, and throw it all over, the Dish. Says she, take good Gravy, according to the Bigness of your Sourtout, some Truffles, Morels, Mushrooms, a Sweet-

bread

bread cut to Pieces, Artichoke-bottoms cut fmall,
and let all ftew together. She adds, take the Yolks
of two or three Eggs, according as you want them,
beat them up with White-wine, ftir altogether one
Way; when it is thick, let it cool, and pour it into
the Surtout: Take the Yolks of a few hard Eggs,
Mace, Pepper, and Salt; and after all, cover it all
over with Force-meat; rub the Yolks all over to
collar, and fend it to an Oven: And, fhe fays, Half
an Hour will do it. This Surtout, to me, looks
fomething like a Force-meat Puff-pafte Pye, dreffed
very cunningly, contrived as the Force-meat is laid
round the Difh: And as this Teacher fays, cover it
with Force-meat; fo Reafon would think, that
the Time that this Force-meat required baking,
would be fufficient to bake the Snipes; for the
Bread, Suet, Herbs, and other Ingredients will not
roll out fo thin as Puff-pafte, very far from it: Then
who in common Reafon would order the Guts to
be pulled out of Snipes, and to half roaft them, and
then to bake them. I've feen a Wager on the
Weight of a Snipe, that it would not weigh two
Ounces, which it did not.

Next, the Teacher gives Orders *to boil Snipes or
Woodcocks:* Says fhe, boil them in good ftrong
Broth, or Beef-gravy made thus: So fummons a
a large Collection of Beef, Onions, Herbs, Mace,
Cloves, Pepper; and while the Snipes are boiling,
ftew the Guts and Livers, with Part of the Gravy
the Snipes are boiled in. In my Opinion, this Lady
Teacher pronounces double Deftruction to Snipes
and Woodcocks: Firft, in Surtout: Secondly, in
boiling them in fuch Variety of Mixtures, to rob
them of their natural Tafte; the moft efteemed tame
Fowl may be fometimes mafqueraded in Cookery,
where they are more plentiful: But wild Fowl are
Rarities, that be very ill to catch hold of at fome
Seafons of the Year, and in their natural Shapes
grace

grace every Table; and a Dinner is very feldom thought elegant that has not wild Fowl plain roafted. This Teacher puts great Hardfhips on the ignorant Maids, by giving them very unneceffary Trouble; but far greater, the Impofition on their Mafters, whofe Fortunes fuffer greatly by Extravagance; and if they eat thofe odd Mixtures and Jumbles, they will confume Health as faft as their Wealth.

In Page 97, To fcare a Hare. This Teacher bids lard your Hare, and put a Pudding in her Belly; and then put her in a Pot or Fifh-kettle, with two Quarts of ftrong draw'd Gravy, one of Red-wine, a Lemon cut, a Faggot of Sweet-herbs, Nutmeg, Pepper, Salt, and Cloves; to ftew till it be three Parts done; then it is to be taken out of the Liquor and put into a Difh, and ftrewed over with Crumbs of Bread, chopt Sweet-herbs, grated Lemon-peel, and half a Nutmeg; to be boiled and brown'd before the Fire: Then fays fhe, in the mean Time take the Fat of the Gravy, and thicken it with the Yolk of an Egg; take fix boil'd hard Eggs chopt fmall, fome pickled Cucumbers cut thin; mix thefe with the Sauce, and pour into the Difh. But I fay, that a Quart of Wine would intoxicate a Man, much more a Hare, my only Favourite: I like the Hare fo well, that I am very angry to fee her fo much abufed; for I never robb'd her of her natural Tafte, but fhewed the Art of Cookery in preferving it: How many Mixtures, and what various Colours, Red, White, Green, and Yellow Sauce, and Extravagance to a Degree.

She adds, that a Fillet of Mutton, or Neck of Venifon, may be done the fame Way. And if a Fillet of the largeft Mutton weighs a Pound, it exceeds the Weight of any I ever faw: Now, I think, fhe fhould have told the Illiterate what Part of the Mutton fhe calls the Fillet (if fhe knows it herfelf:) The Fillet is the Collop that lies in the Infide of the

the Loin of Mutton, next to the Chain; and if the ignorant Maid has of herself found it out, it will not be to her Master's Profit.

Although her Mistress says, that you may do Rabbits the same Way. But instead of Beef, it must be Veal-gravy; and the Red-wine turned into White-wine, adding Cucumbers for Mushrooms.

Page 98, She stews a Hare with as many Mixtures; but does not intoxicate her so extravagantly with Wine, prescribing only one Spoonful.

Next is, *A Hare Civet.* She bids bone the Hare, and take out the Sinews; then cut one Half into thin Slices, and the other Half in Pieces an Inch thick; to flour and fry them in Butter like Collops quick, and to have ready some good Gravy made of the Hare's Bones and Beef; put a Pint of it into a Pan to the Hare, a little Mustard and Elder-vinegar; to stew it till it be as thick as Cream.

This Teacher has no Connection with the true Art of Cookery: For strong Meat, as Pork, Beef, or Goose, Mustard and Vinegar, may help Digestion, and is very proper: But the harmless Hare that never gave Offence to any Stomach, except such Cookery as this Teacher has prescribed to the Hare.

Her next is, *Portuguese Rabbits.* I have, says she, in the Beginning of my Book, given Directions for Boiled and Roasted. Get some Rabbits, truss them Chicken Fashion; their Heads must be cut off, and the Rabbits turned with their Back upwards, and two of the Legs stripped to the Claw-end, and so trussed with two Skewers: Lard and roast them with what Sauce you please. If you want Chickens, and they are to appear as such, they must be dress'd in this Manner: Or if they are to be boiled for Chickens, cut off their Heads, and cover them with white Sellery-sauce, or Rice-sauce, tossed up with Cream, says she.

When I see this Teacher's Transformation of
Rabbits

Rabbits into Chickens, it raifed me from very low
to high Spirits ; being but newly recovered from a
long Sicknefs, which had funk my Spirits very low,
till *Portuguefe* Rabbits raifed them to their full
Height : When I faw how eafy it was to the Teacher to make Rabbits into Chickens, no more than cut
off their Heads, turn up their Backs, and ftrip the
two Legs to the Claw-end, and fo trufs'd with two
Skewers. I thought myfelf in the Midft of an Affembly of illiterate Maids ; every one had a Rabbit
trying their utmoft Skill to make a Chicken of the
four footed Creature ; fome ftripped the Fore-legs
to the Claw-end ; fome the Hind-legs ; but none of
them could make the Links of the Back ply into
the Form of a Chicken Breaft : And by the Strength
of Imagination, I thought I heard the whole Pupil
Affembly give their Teacher a general Curfe for af-
firming her Art of Cookery eafy ; which by Trial
they found impracticable, and her Transformation a
mere Cheat on their Underftandings.

Next is, *A Rabbit Surprize.* To roaft two half
grown Rabbits ; you muft cut off their Heads and
firft Joints ; then tofs the Lean of the Back-bones
with Cream and Butter, till it is thick and good ;
and then upon the Back-bone of each Rabbit is a
long Trough of Force-meat to be fix'd, and filled
with the tofs'd up Flefh that is taken of the roafted
Rabbits Backs, which is to be cover'd with Force-
meat, rubb'd over with raw Egg ; make your Troughs
fquare at each End, and to be baked three Qua-
ters of an Hour. Query, Whether fhe gave the
Force-meat a proper Foundation, to fecure the Gravy
or Cream-fauce from being let out by the Back-
links of the Rabbits? or let it be double and treble
Query'd, whether ever Troughs were built on Rabbits Backs before? If the Lady's Ingenuity enables
her to metamorphize Rabbits into Chickens, and
build large fquare ended Troughs on their Back, no
doubt

doubt but through the Profoundity of her Contrivances, she'll be finding out the Mystery of transforming them to Elephants, and erecting Forcemeat Castles on their Backs.

In Page 100, *is a Neck of Mutton*, call'd *The hasty Dish*. This Teacher bids take a large Pewter or Silver Dish, with an Edge about an Inch deep on the Inside, on which the Lid fixes, with a Handle at Top, so fast that you may lift it up full by the Handle without falling; this Dish is called a Necromancer: She bids take a Neck of Mutton of six Pounds, cut into Chops, a sliced *French* Roll, a large Onion, four Turnips, a Bundle of Sweet-herbs, three Blades of Mace; all these are to be put into this Dish, in their separate Lairs, and to fill it with boiling Water, and cover it close; to hang the Dish on the Backs of two Chairs by the Rim; to tear three Sheets of brown Paper into fifteen Pieces, which are to be drawn through your Hand; light one Piece of Paper, and hold it under the Bottom of your Dish, moving the Paper about, and as fast as one burns light another, till all is burnt, and your Meat will be enough; fifteen Minutes just does it: This Dish, says she, was first contrived by Mr. *Rich*, and is much admired by the Nobility. Very likely Mr. *Rich* might be on his Travels in a very poor Country, where there might be great Scarcity of firing and good Cooks; so Necessity, the Mother of Invention, might produce the above Contrivance to get Support on the Road: But will Reason, or the least Art of Cookery dictate, that the Flame of three Sheets of Paper will boil six Pounds of Mutton cut into Chops, with Turnips, Onions, Herbs, &c. notwithstanding the boiling Water she orders at first to be poured on the Meat, &c. The very Quantity of Flesh, Herbs, &c. will so much abate the Heat of the Water, that to me it seems very unreasonable, that such a small Force of Heat, as can proceed from
three

three fired Sheets, will never make her Meat and Broth to boil; and if fuch Cookery amounts to a tolerable fcald, 'tis as much as any reafonable Perfon might expect, unlefs there be more Heat and Strength in Paper than my Imagination dictates, Trial muft be allowed the beft Proof: And whoever has a-mind to be befool'd into fuch a ridiculous Experiment, have my free Leave; as for my Part, I fhall not make an *April* Idiot of myfelf, nor perfwade any of my Readers thereto. If this Inventor, Mr. *Rich*, be Mr. *Rich*, the famous Harlequin and Mafter-player, at the *New Theatre, Covent Garden*; it may not be altogether impoffible, but that he might put fuch a Pun on the Lady Teacher, and fuch others of her Pretenfions, that have laboured hard to impofe on their Betters, by calling black white, fweet bitter, bitter fweet, unwholefome wholefome, *&c.* Query, whether a Perfon going haftily by might not with their Cloths move one of the Chairs, or a Dog being in the Room, pufhing by or through the Chairs, would not bring down this fine Invention in the Twinkling of an Eye?

Page 102, *Another Way to make a Pellow.* Take a Leg of Veal of twelve or fourteen Pounds Weight, and an old Cock skinned; chop both to Pieces, and put into a Pot with fix Blades of Mace, fome whole White-pepper, and three Gallons of Water, half a Pound of Bacon, two Onions and fix Cloves; cover it clofe, and when it boils let it do very foftly, till the Meat is good for nothing, and above two Thirds wafted, then ftrain it; the next Day put this Soop into a Sauce-pan, with a Pound of Rice, fet it over a flow Fire, take Care it don't burn; when the Rice is thick and dry, turn into a Difh. Garnifh with hard Eggs cut in two; and have roafted Fowls in another Difh.

By the Rice and Eggs in one Difh, and the roafted Fowls in another; in all likelihood the Teacher

E   designs defigns the thick dry Rice and hard Egg-fauce, for the roafted Fowls; but whoever gets the Rice in their Mouths, 'twill ftick to their Teeth like Bird-lime; for the old Cock muft weigh at leaft four Pounds, and fourteen of Veal; fo that the Strength of eighteen Pounds of Meat to a Pound of Rice, will make it of fo glutonous a Nature, that whoever has it in their Mouths, will find it ftick fo clofe, that they'll be thankful to have it out again; fo there is wafted what would have made feven Difhes of Meat.—I divide the Veal into four Parts; five Pounds I cut to the Knockel, and boil with Greens and the half Pound of Bacon; then I cut four Pounds to the Fillet, and this I make a Ragoo of; and of three Pounds I make a Difh of *Scotch* Collops; and two Pounds I *A-la-mond*; and the Gravy of the Knockel will be Sauce for the Made Difhes; and of the Pound of Rice and hard Eggs, I make two Rice-puddings, the one baked and the other boil'd; then, inftead of the old Cock, I take a young Pout, (which may be as eafily purchafed in the Market as an old one) this I roaft, with Egg-fauce: So far Teachers differ in their Opinions in Cookery; for as the Cock, Bacon, and Veal are to boil till the Meat be good for nothing; and as the Rice was ordered, it was good for nothing; fo I make feven Difhes of Meat out of nothing, by the Lady Teacher's nothing arian Ingenuity.

Next is, *Effence of Ham.* Take the Fat off the Ham, and cut the Lean in Slices; beat them well, and lay them in the Bottom of a Stew-pan, with Slices of Carrots, Parfnips, and Onions; let them ftew over a gentle Fire till they begin to ftick; then fprinkle a little Flour, and turn them; then moiften with Broth and Veal-gravy; feafon them with three or four Mufhrooms, as many Truffles, a whole Leak, or a Clove of Garlick, fome Parfley, and half a Dozen of Cloves; put in fome Crufts of

Bread,

Bread, and let them fimmer over the Fire for a Quarter of an Hour; ftrain it, and fet it away for Ufe. Any Pork or Ham does for this, that is well made.

Thus far the Lady directs, thofe who do not know the right Way, are apt to take the Wrong, fay I: For this Teacher reminds me of the Fable of the Hen that laid the golden Eggs every Day; but the covetous Owner not being fatisfied, cut up the Hen to catch all at once; but he pay'd dear for his covetous Search, lofing all; even fo has this Teacher done the golden Effence of Ham, by cutting it in Pieces, although fhe keeps the Drofs for Ufe, which is only fit to give to Dogs. And as an Inftance of her fine judicious Tafte of Ham Effence; fhe fays, any Pork Ham does for this Ufe; and fo far I hold with her, for any Thing of that Kind is too good to wafte; but that the Difference of Tafte between new and old Ham Effence, is as widely different, as is the Tafte of good old Beer, and New in the working Fat. Now the Difference between the Teacher's Effence, and the true Effence of Ham is this: I take a two Years old Ham, wafhes it in hot Water with a coarfe Cloth; then lays it in warm Water four Hours, and afterwards puts it into a large Pot in cold Water, makes a brisk Fire to it, and when it is boiled enough, I take it up and run it through in feveral Places with an Iron Skewer, and the Gravy that runs from it, is the true Effence; and this Gravy put into Jelly-glaffes hot, the Fat that iffues out along with the Gravy will be as a Seal to preferve the Effence, and it will keep fix Months, and the Ham will ftill remain very palatable; although I can't but acknowledge, that a Ham ought to go to the Table full of its Juice, if you would have it in its Perfection; but, as I above obferved, it will ftill remain Taftable, and be a very good cold Relifh.

Next,

Next, the Teacher's *Rules to be observed in all Made Dishes*; Are, that all White-sauces have a little Tartness, smooth, and of a fine Thickness; and that all the Time the Sauces are over the Fire, keep stirring them one Way: And that Brown-sauces are not to swim with Fat on the Top, but to be smooth, and as thick as good Cream, and not to taste of one Thing more than of another; and as to Pepper and Salt, season to your Palate; but don't put too much of either Sort, left you take away the fine Flavour of every Thing: And as to most Made Dishes, you may put in what you think proper, to enrich or make it good, as pickel'd Mushrooms, Cocks-combs, Ox-palates, Artichoke-bottoms, Asparagus, &c.

Here the Lady leaves her Pupils in a Wood, and to their own wild Imaginations; so that their Cookery may as probably be vitiated as made wholsome, by young Beginners in the Art of Cookery; and as to the judicious Cook, she might as well have remained silent; and if the bare reading these, and such like her Rules compleat the House-wife, Cookery will be very easily attained. And here I differ in my Judgment with the Lady's ordering Sauces to be stirred but one Way, all the Time they are on the Fire; for the perfect experienced Cook has many various Methods in tossing and turning Sauces; and for her Brown-sauce to be as thick as good Cream, then will a Spoon stand upright in the Sauce; and as to her Seasoning to the Palate, if the illiterate Cook be void of Palate and Judgment; then she may copy after her Teacher, by heaping in all Rarities at once, without regard to Quantity, Weight, or Measure, doing all at Random, hit or miss, Luck's all.

In Page 103, This Lady Teacher bids *read this Chapter, and you will find how expensive French Cook Sauce is*: Wherein is contained two Sauces, *viz.* Essence of Ham, and five Cullisses. Partridge Sauce, she calls, an odd Jumble of Trash; and when all the

Ingredients

Ingredients are reckoned, the Partridge will come to a fine Penny of Money.

A Cullis for all Sorts of Ragoo: This she bids compute the Expence, and see if this Dish cannot be dressed full as well without this Expence.

Cullis the Italian Way: To which she says, now this *Italian*, or *French*-sauce is saucy. Concludes with, they will make as many fine Ingredients to stew a Pigeon or Fowl, as would make a very fine Dish; which is equal with boiling a Leg of Mutton in Champain; and adds, it would be needless to name any more, though you have much more expensive Sauce than this: However, she thinks here is enough to shew the Folly of the fine *French* Cooks. She says, in their own Country, they will make a grand Entertainment with the Expence of one of these Dishes; but here they want the little petty Profit, and by such Sort of Legerdemain, some fine Estates are jugled into *France*. By these Aspersions the Lady Teacher gives the *French* Cooks, it may be supposed, that her great Fortune has been impaired by the Extravagancy of a *French* Cook; for in this Lady's Preface, she says, if Gentlemen will have *French* Cooks, they must pay for *French* Tricks, and seems to be grieved at the blind Folly of the Age; says, they would rather be imposed on by a *French* Booby, than give Encouragement to a good *English* Cook. It appears to me, that the Lady builds her Monument of Fame upon the Ruins she makes of the *French* Cooks Characters: I don't like the Foundation she has chosen; for notwithstanding all her great Bravadoes of Thrift, she has tenfold more extravavagant *French* Cookery in her Book, then in the Chapter she bids you read. As to her first Charge of Partridge Sauce, it comes far short of her Partridge *à la Braise*; and as to the *French* Cooks Essence of Ham, which she has placed in that Chapter for Extravagance; that very individual Essence of Ham,

the

ſhe has in the very Page before; therefore I ſee no Reaſon why it ſhould be a Mark of Infamy on the *French* Cook, and a Trophy of Honour to her.

The French Cooks Cullis for all Sorts of Ragoo : She bids, compute the Expence, and ſee if this Diſh cannot be dreſſed full as well without. I have at her Requeſt made a Computation, and cannot juſtly make the Charge amount to above two Shillings, and that exceeds the Thrift of her Preface Cullis, which ſhe braves them with; yet this *French* Cullis for all Sorts of Ragoo, is one Shilling cheaper than that very thrifty Preface Cullis is.

Now her ſecond Chapter, which this Teacher calls *Made Diſhes*. I have not ſeen a Book of Cookery yet printed, that ſhe has not plundered to make up this Chapter, which contains Two hundred and thirty Diſhes and upwards. And although ſhe ſeems to have been a great Traveller by the Cookery preſcribed from different Nations, *viz. Turkey, Germany, Portugal,* and *India* ; yet put all the Cookery ſhe quotes from them together, ſhe has twenty *French* Diſhes in this Chapter to each one Diſh of all the ſeparate Nations.

I think ſhe has made publick Demonſtration of the Regard ſhe pays to *French* Cooks, by engroſſing ſo many of their Diſhes of Surfeits and Inconſiſtencies in her Chapter; that ſhe had not left a ſufficient Number to make out the eight expenſive Sauces, till ſhe broke Bulk for Eſſence of Ham, and was ſo pinched as to charge them with *Italian* Extravagance, or take more out of her own Chapter. As to all the *French* Cookery I ever ſee in Print, I thought it a Burleſque upon the *Engliſh,* whom they ſay would exceed all the World for Wiſdom if they did not eat ſuch groſs Food: And as there was but little Regard taken of their Preſcriptions, 'tis poſſible that it was generally looked on in the ſame Light.

Yet this Lady Teacher has artfully abuſed the
French

French Cooks, and as cunningly recommended their
Cookery for her own; fo by what fhe collects from
them and other Authors, fhe becomes Miftrefs of
the Art, and fays fhe has made it plain and eafy,
concluding her Preface with; fhe hopes her Book
will anfwer the Ends fhe intended it for, which are
to improve the Servants, and fave the Ladies a great
deal of Trouble. And begins her firft Chapter by
faying, that profeft Cooks will find Fault with touching upon a Branch of Cookery, which they never
thought worth their Notice, is what I expect, &c.
And adds, that fhe does not pretend to teach profefs'd Cooks, but defigns to inftruct the ignorant
and unlearned, (which will likewife be of great Ufe
in all private Families) and in fo plain and full a Manner, that the moft illiterate and ignorant Perfon,
who can but read, will know how to do every
Thing in Cookery well.

A noble Pennyworth in Cookery, if this Teacher
has performed the publick Promifes of the Benefits
the Ignorant and Unlearned fhould receive by the
reading her Book: But if not, it was a Puff to help
the Sale of it, as fhe could not give them the Knowledge fhe has not herfelf, nor ever will poffefs it.
Therefore muft be a double Impofition: Firft, In
deluding and depriving the Ladies of their Healths.
Secondly, In caufing the ignorant Servants to throw
away their Money, and filling them full of vain
Glory. Now, if there is fuch a fovereign Virtue in
the naked reading of her Book, without a Capacity
of Underftanding, which poffibly cannot be in the
Ignorant: Then which Way does every ignorant
Maid arrive to fuch an exalted Pitch of Knowledge
in Cookery, as to do every Thing therein well:
Why might fhe not as well pretend to teach profef-
fed Cooks? For it is my Opinion, that the Univerfe
cannot produce that Cook who knows how to do
every Branch in Cookery well. Does not every feparate

parate Nation produce fomething that their Neighbours want, and differ in their various Ways of
Cookery? And let a Cook fearch into thofe Arts,
and be his Genius as great as poffible, if he fays he
can do all Cookery well, I will not believe him. I
have a Circumftance of Error to produce, which I
can affirm for Truth, that a Houfe-keeper to a Perfon of Diftinction, robb'd the Sirloin of the Infide
of the Fillet of Beef, the moft delicious Part of the
four Quarters; which fhe took for a Made Difh, and
fent up the Sirloin to the Table with the Out-fide;
but no In-fide was there, which is the Favourite of
all Beef Eaters: Some Gentlemen being then at Dinner, and who were difappointed of their favourite
Piece of roaft Beef, put the Lady to the Blufh; who
enquired of her Houfe-keeper, the Reafon of her
fending to the Table fuch a naked Sirloin of Beef:
She anfwered her Lady, that fhe made a fine Difh of
the Fillet; but, (anfwers the Lady) you have fpoil'd
a much finer, and therefore I difcharge you for ever
to commit the fame Fault. Yet, notwithftanding,
this Houfe-keeper prepoffeft in favour of, and de-
pending upon the Infallibity of her Lady Teacher;
and as her Lady Miftrefs was but young, confidered
which of thefe two Ladies fhe owed moft Duty to;
and after an inward doubting, gave her Teacher the
Preference, who had given her full Affurance of doing every Thing in Cookery well. So fhe cuts off
the Fillet a fecond Time, and fent up a naked Sirloin to the Table; for which fhe got her Difcharge,
loft a good Place, and fhed Floods of Tears for her
vain Glory; for which fhe might thank her Lady
Teacher. This plainly demonftrates, that the Age
is not fo blind, as that all are to be impofed upon by
the Follies of this celebrated Lady Teacher. The
Wifdom of the young Lady, Miftrefs of her Houfe
fhows, in turning off her Servant, both for wafting
her Meat, and difobeying her Orders. And if thefe
are

are the **Teacher's** promifed Benefits to the Ignorant, fhe cheats them both of their Money and Places; and inftead of faving the Ladies a great deal of Trouble, teaches their Cooks to prepare fuch Surfeits as may give them Pain.

In Page 107, *Is to force Hogs Ears:* This Teacher fays, the Ears are to be boiled, and a Force-meat to be made; to flit the Ears very carefully to make a Place for your Stuffing; fhe bids alfo fill and flour them, fry them; then ftew them in Wine, Muftard, Pepper, Onion and Gravy: Difh them up and pour on the Sauce.

It feems very eafy to the Teacher, to bid flit the Hogs Ears very carefully to make a Place for the Stuffing; yet it is out of her Power to divide the Griffel of thefe Ears to fill them with Force-meat; and when fhe has made the beft of them fhe can, fhe will not make filken Purfes of her Hogs Ears.

Next is, *To force Cocks-combs:* Parboil your Cockscombs, fays fhe; then open them with the Point of a Knife at the Great-end; then take the White of a Fowl, as much Bacon and Beef-marrow, beat in a Mortar, with an Egg and Seafoning, to fill the Cocks-combs, and ftew them in Gravy.

So fmall is the Morfel that grows on the Crown of the Cocks Heads, that the Stuffing this Teacher has ordered to be made, all the Cocks-combs in *England,* opened at the Great-end, will not have Room to hold it. The Morfel is an Ornament in Made Difhes; but where to find Room for Stuffing in that fmall Matter, is the Query.

Next fhe tells, *How to preferve Cocks-combs:* To put them into a Pot with melted Bacon, and let them boil half an Hour; add Bay-falt, Pepper, Vinegar, fliced Lemon, and an Onion ftuck with Cloves: When the Bacon begins to ftick to the Pot, to take them up, and put them into the Pan, and pour

F   clari-

clarified Butter over them: Thefe, fays fhe, make a pretty Plate at Supper.

This Teacher bids boil the fmall Morfels of Cocks-combs in melted Bacon half an Hour: A fufficient Time indeed to burn them to as many black Cinders; and after the many other Ingredients are added, *viz.* Vinegar, fliced Lemon, Onion, Cloves; and thefe, fays fhe, makes a pretty Difh for Supper. The above-mentioned are the Product of this Teacher's own Cookery, but preferv'd Cocks-combs fets forth the Truth of her Art of Cookery; for, after the Cocks-combs have boiled half an Hour in Bacon; a little Vinegar, and the fliced Lemon are to be put into the boiling Fat, which would give a Crack like a Cannon; fo that there would be no need of the Chimney fweeping; for the Blaft would bring down the Soot at once, and deftroy the pretty Supper-plate; although the Teacher had taken a Method to blaft the Beauty, by the half Hour's boiling, in the Bacon-fat.

In Page 112, *A forced Cabbage:* Take a White-heart Cabbage, as big as a Quarter of a Peck, half boil it, and cut out the Heart, but take Care not to break off any of the out-fide Leaves; to make a Force-meat of a Pound of Veal, half a Pound of Ham, four hard Eggs, Herbs and Seafonings; Mufhrooms and the Cabbage-coftick chopt amongft the Reft finely, all mixt with the Yolk of an Egg, and put into the hollow Part of the Cabbage, tie it with Pack-thread; Slices of Bacon are to be laid on the Bottom of a Stew-pan, upon which is a Pound of Beef cut thin to be laid, and the Cabbage to be laid above all clofe: 'Tis to be covered and fet to ftew over a Fire till the Bacon fticks to the Pan; then, fays fhe, fhake Flour and pour in a Quart of Broth, Onion, Cloves, Mace, White-pepper, a Bundle of Sweet-herbs; clofe cover it, and let it ftew an Hour and an Half; then put in a Glafs of Red-wine, and give

give it a boil; then, says she, take it up and lay it in the Dish, and strain the Gravy over, untie it first. This, says she, is a fine Dish, and the next Day makes a fine Hash, with a Veal Stake nicely broiled and laid on it.

In my Opinion, this forced Cabbage would be a Hash the first Day; which would give all Stomachs that receiv'd it such a Disgust, as would make them say, from Cabbage-costick, Force-meat, *Good Lord deliver us!*

In Page 125, *Is a White Peas Soop*: Wherein the Teacher bids, take three Pounds of thick Flank of Beef, half a Pound of Bacon, a Bundle of Sweet-herbs, and a good Quantity of dry'd Mint, a Bunch of the green Tops of Sellery, a Quart of split Peas, and three Gallons of Water, to be close covered, and set on the Fire, and let it boil till two Parts are wasted; then to be strained, and six Heads of Sellery cut small and put in it, to boil to three Quarts; then cut fat and lean Bacon, and Bread into Dices, and fry'd; to season the Soop with Salt, and rub dry'd Mint over, after it is poured into the Dish, and so send it to the Table: She says, you may add Force-meat Balls fry'd, Cocks-combs boil'd in it, an Ox's Palate stewed tender and small.

The Teacher sets forth, *Another Way to make it:* She says, when you boil a Leg of Pork, or a good Piece of Beef, save the Liquor: The next Day boil a Leg of Mutton, save the Liquor, when it is cold take off the Fat, and set it on the Fire with two Quarts of Peas, let them boil till they are tender; then put in the Pork and Beef Liquor, with the In-gredients as above, and let it boil till it be as thick as you would have it, allowing for the boiling. A-gain, says she, strain it off, and add the Ingredients as above. Likewise, you may make your Soop of Veal, or Mutton-gravy, if you please, that is according to your Fancy.

None

None boils a Leg of Pork before it is firſt ſalted; ſo it is as common to ſalt Beef, the Broth of which very few Gentry will let their Servants eat; but to make a Peas Soop withal. The Ingredients which this Lady has cram'd into the above, and the under Soop, ſcarce any Dog's Stomach, I think, is able to digeſt; or if it could, it would certainly throw them into ſome Leproſy: The firſt Time I peruſed this Soop, I loathed Meat for three Days.

In Page 127, *To make Hodge-podge:* To which ſhe takes a Pound of Beef, a Pound of Veal, and a Pound of a Scraig of Mutton cut into little Pieces; to be ſet on the Fire with two Quarts of Water, an Ounce of Barley, Onion, Sweet-herbs, four Heads of Sellery, Mace, Cloves, Whole-pepper, three Turnips, one Carrot, two Lettices cut ſmall; put all in the Pot, and let it ſtew ſoftly over a ſlow Fire five or ſix Hours; take out the Spice, Herbs, and Onion, and pour all into a Soop-diſh.

I think there would be no Manner of Occaſion for a Soop-diſh, nor any Broth to pour into it: It would be a Wonder if the three Pounds of Meat, Barley, Roots, and other Ingredients, were not burnt to the Pot-bottom, let it ſtew ever ſo ſlowly; for two Quarts will not ſtand five or ſix Hours ſimmering without being exhauſted dry, if not burnt to the Pot-bottom, as the Lady has preſcribed.

In Page 128, *Is a Portable Soop:* This Teacher bids, take two Legs of Beef, of fifty Pounds Weight, and take off all the Skin and Fat, and take the Meat and Sinews clean from the Bones; which Meat put into a large Pot with eight or nine Gallons of Water. She bids, add to it twelve Anchovies, Mace, and Pepper, each an Ounce, Cloves, a Quarter of an Ounce, ſix large Onions, a Bundle of Sweet-herbs, the Cruſt of a Two-penny Loaf; ſtir all together, cover it cloſe, and lay a Weight on the Cover; and when it has boiled eight or nine

Hours

Hours uncover it, and ftir it altogether; cover it a-
gain, and let it boil till it becomes a rich good Jelly.
She fays, when you think it is a thick jelly, take it
off and ftrain it through a coarfe Hair-bag, prefs it
hard; then ftrain it through a Hair-fieve into a large
Earthen-pan; when it is quite cold take off the Skim
and Fat, and take the fine Jelly clear from the Settlings.

Now for a good Wager, I could venture to make
more Glue of the Bones and Sinews, which this
Teacher feparates from the Meat of two fifty Pound
Legs of Beef, then fhe fhall do with the Meat and
all hot Spices, Anchovies, &c. which to me is poi-
foning any Soop. Portable Soop was contrived to
fupport tender Travellers on the Road; but what
Support can reafonably be left in the Lady's Glue?
for the Skin, Fat, Bones, and Sinews taken from
the Meat, as the Teacher terms it; fo that fhe leaves
as much of the two Legs as fhe takes; to which
nine Gallons of Water are to boil eight or nine
Hours; a fufficient Time for all the Strength and
Tafte of the Meat to fteam out in Smoak and Air;
yet it will take fixteen Hours to bring this Meat
to fo thick a Jelly, by flow boiling; and the Cruft
of a Two-penny Loaf, boiling fo long a Time in the
Broth, muft make it thick, after preffing the Jelly fo
hard through a coarfe Hair-bag: Although, fhe bids,
ftrain it through a Hair-fieve into a large Earthen-
pan; and when cold, to take off the fine Jelly clear
from the Settlings Now, I put the Query, how
this fine Jelly gets clear from the Cruft of the Two-
penny Loaf? becaufe boiling fo long it would become a Pafte-glue, rather than a clear Jelly; which
this Teacher makes manifeft, in boiling it afterwards
in a well tin'd Stew-pan; which, fhe bids, take
great Care that it neither ftick to the Pan or burn,
as it will be Lumps about the Pan; which Lumps
are to be put into China-cups fet into Water and
boiled;

boiled; and when the Glue is cool turn it on coarse Flannel; let it lie eight or nine Hours, keep it in a warm dry Place, and turn it on fresh Flannel till it be quite dry, and the Glue will be quite hard. I think the Method which this Teacher prescribes to dry this Glue, must be dangerous to the Stomach; for it would pull all the Wool from off the coarse new Flannels, and by turning it on fresh Flannel till it become quite dry, the Wool would be so interwoven with the Glue, as to make a sad Spectacle, as well as a dangerous Prescription of it: And as the Teacher has not given Orders to strain the Gravy when the Glue was melted, it is very doubtful that those who have supp'd most of her Soop, must eat most Wool. Now, the Teacher bids, when you use it to pour boiling Water on it, and keep it stirring all the Time till it be melted: She says, a Piece as big as a large Walnut will make a Pint of Water very rich: And further the Lady directs, how to make Soops and strong Sauces of this Glue; and says, this is only in the Room of a rich good Gravy. Yet I will give any of her Adherents all this rich Glue, that she has made of her two fifty Pound Legs of Beef directed; and for a Wager will make a better Soop of five Pounds of Beef, with only the Help of Roots.

In Page, 130: This Teacher bids bake an *Oat Pudding:* She says, of Oats decoticated, take two Pounds, and of new Milk enough to drown it, and eight Ounces of Rasins stoned, an equal Quantity of Currans neatly pick'd, a Pound of Sweet-suet finely shred, six new-laid Eggs well beat; season with Nutmeg, Ginger, and Salt: This, says she, will make a better Pudding than Rice. But I say that Rice is far superior to half-sheel'd Oats for Puddings, nor would I advise any to eat this Oat Pudding that has a sore Throat, for the Seeds would certainly give them great Pain.

Her

Her next is, *A Calf's Foot Pudding:* Take of Calves Feet a Pound minced fine, a Pound and a Half of Suet shred small, six Eggs, but half the Whites, the Crumb of a Half-penny Roll grated, a Pound of Currans, and a Handful of Flour, as much Milk as will moisten it with the Eggs, Salt, Nutmeg, and Sugar; season it to your Taste, and boil it, says she, nine Hours with your Meat.

What is there in this Pudding that can endure nine Hours boiling; the Calves Feet must be tender boil'd, or they will not mince fine; the small shred Suet needs very little boiling, the Handful of Flour, the Crumbs of the Half-penny Loaf grated, Eggs, Fruit and all together, seems to me not to require above an Hour's boiling; and if it boils Nine, what will it be then, or what Limb of the Bullock can stand nine Hours boiling, and keep whole?

In Page 136, *Is Ham Pye:* The Teacher bids, take some cold boil'd Ham, and slice it about half an Inch thick, to make a good Crust, and thick, over the Dish, and lay a Lair of Ham, shake Pepper over it; then lay a large young Fowl on the Ham, with Yolks of Eggs hard boil'd; and cover all with Ham, and more Pepper to be shaked on; then put on the Top-crust; bake it well, and when it comes out of the Oven, fill it with rich Beef-gravy: Adds, that a fresh Ham will not be so tender: So, says she, I always boil my Ham one Day and bring it to Table, the next Day I make a Pye of it: It does better than an unboil'd Ham.

But, I say, the Teacher might as reasonably say, that a Leg of Mutton should be first boil'd, and the next Day made into a Pye, as to boil the Ham, and then to bake it: As to her own she might order it her own Way, but when her Orders are general, her Judgment should have been better in Ham Pye making.

In

[48]

In Page 193, *Is to make a Yorkshire Christmas Pye:*
A Bushel of Flour is to be made into a standing
Crust; which according to her Directions in *Page*
145, for *Standing Crusts* will take 24 Pounds of Butter; a Turkey, Goose, Fowl, Partridge, and a Pigeon, are to be boned, and put one within another, and all to be put into a large Turkey; Black-
pepper, Nutmeg, and Mace of each half an Ounce,
Cloves a quarter of an Ounce, two Spoonfuls of Salt;
this great Turkey is laid in the Crust, to look like a
whole one; then is a Hare cut to Pieces, and laid
on one Side; on the other Side Woodcocks, Moor-
game, and what Sort of wild Fowl you can get:
All to be seasoned well, and laid close; four Pounds
of Butter at least is to be put into this Pye, and a
very thick Lid to be laid on; and it must, says she,
have a very hot Oven, and will take at least four
Hours baking.

I should think that a Pye with such a Crust, and
so well filled, would take fourteen Hours, if the
Walls stood; which in my Opinion is impossible, for
the great Quantity of Butter she orders her standing Crusts without Water, or as little as you can
when you skim it off, says she; so this greasy Crust
so well filled, and four Pounds of Butter put over
all, must make such a Stench in the Oven, as would
bring down the Pye; and if it was set whole into
the Oven, it must come out in Parcels; and I think
I could make a Corporation Feast of the Expence
of this *Yorkshire Christmas* Pye.

In Page 144, *is Paste for Tarts.* Take one Pound
of Flour, three Quarters of a Pound of Butter; mixt
and beat well with a Rolling-pin.

Another Sort of *Paste* for *Tarts,* which is Butter,
Flour, and Sugar, of each half a Pound; mixt and
well beat with a Rolling-pin, and then roll it out.

But, I say, the half Pound of Flour is so far out-
match'd with the Sugar and Butter, that the ignorant

unt Girl must exceed me in Pastry, if she can roll
out a Lid for a Tart, as she is directed by her
Teacher.

In Page 145, is a Dripping Crust: She orders a
Pound and a Half of Beef-drippings to be boil'd up
five Times in Water, and set to cool; then to work
it up well in three Pounds of Flour as fine as you
can, and make it up into Paste with cold Water:
It makes a very fine Crust, says she, of the Sort. Say
I, which Sort I would not willingly recommend to
delicate Ladies Stomachs.

Next follows A Crust for Custards: Take eight
Ounces of Flour, to six Ounces of Butter, three
Spoonfuls of Cream, mix all together, and let them
stand a Quarter of an Hour; then work it up and
down, and roll it thin. For my Part, I cannot find
out the meaning of this up and down Custard Crust.

And next is, Paste for Crackling Crusts. This Crust
is to be made of four Handfuls of Almonds, throw
them into Water, dry them with a Cloth, and pound
them in a Mortar very fine, with a little Orange-
flower-water, and the White of an Egg; all to be well
pounded, and put through a coarse Hair-sieve, to
clear them from all the Lumps or Clods, says she;
then spread it on a Dish till it is very pliable; let it
stand a while, and then roll out a Piece for the Under-crust, and dry it in the Oven in the Pye-pan,
while other Pastry-works are a making, as Knots,
Cyphers, &c. for garnishing your Pyes.

This is very odd Pastry-cookery for the Ignorant
to be improv'd by, for their Teacher has left them
in the Dark as to the finishing this Pye, by putting the
Under-crust into the Pye-pan, and setting it in the
Oven to dry; but does not tell them what this Under-crust is to be filled with, or how, or in what
Manner they are to proceed with this Pye: I can
see nothing the designs for it, but Knots and Cyphers for garnishing, to this Under-crust; so I call
it

it a Cypher Pye, which in reality it muſt be; for if there is a Paſtry-cook in *England* that can make this Paſte ſo pliable, (as ſhe calls it) ſo as to raiſe either Tart or Pye, or to turn either out of a Pan, I have loſt my Judgment.

In Page 166, *Is to dreſs a Brace of Carp.* This Teacher bids boil the Carp in Salt and Water; and for Sauce a Pint of ſtale Beer, and a Pint of Red-wine; ſhe adds, Mace, Cloves, Nutmeg, Pepper, O-nion, Sweet-herbs, Anchovy, Horſe-raddiſh, Cat-chup, Muſhroom-pickle, and a Quarter of a Pound of Butter.

Certainly the Pint of Red-wine and the Pint of ſtale Beer boil'd with ſo much hot Spice, would fuddle the Brace of Carp; yet this Teacher has or-dered two baked Carp to be put into a Pan, with a Bottle of White-wine, and as many Ingredients as is above preſcribed.

And, *To fry Tench :* She gives a whole Page of ſuch Inconſiſtences of Cream, Eggs, Bread, Herbs and Spices, Gravy, Wine, &c. &c. and after all, ſays, you may dreſs them juſt as you do Carp.

Next is, *To roaſt a Cod's Head:* The Teacher bids, after the Head is clean waſh'd, to ſalt it and lay it in a Stew-pan before the Fire, with ſomething be-hind it that the Fire may roaſt it; and all the Water that comes from it the firſt half Hour throw away; then ſtrew on Nutmeg, Cloves, Mace, Salt, and Flour; then to be baſted with Butter: When that has lain ſome Time, ſeaſon and flour it, baſte the o-ther Side the ſame Way; turn it often, and baſte it with Crumbs of Bread: If it is a large Head, it will take four or five Hours baking, ſays ſhe; have ready melted Butter, ſome of the Fiſh Liver bruiſed, and an Anchovy mixt well with two Yolks of Eggs; then to be ſtrain'd through a Sieve, and put into the Sauce-pan again; add Shrimps, pickled Cockles, Red-wine, and the Juice of a Lemon; pour it into
the

the Pan the Head was roasted in, and stir it all together, and pour it into the Sauce-pan; keep it stirring, let it boil, and pour it into a Bason: Garnish the Head with fry'd Fish, Lemon, and Horse-raddish.

Five Hours roasting a Cod's Head would make it more fit to grind in a Mill, than to send up to a Lady's Table. The Teacher bids, at the first laying down, to turn it often: It would be a very great Wonder if the ignorant Hand did not turn it out of its natural Shape in four or five Hours; in which Time she did not consider how many Cinders the Pan it was roasted in would catch; nay, the very Crumbs it was basted with would roast to Cinders in that Space of Time; yet has this Teacher bid, pour in all her toss'd-up Sauce into this Pan, and pour it into the Sauce-pan again, and boil it all together; and, I only ask, would not the Yolks of Eggs break the Sauce? But it could not spoil the Head, because that has been done already.

In Page 176, *To broil Haddocks, when they are in high Perfection:* She bids gut and wash them clean, but don't rip open their Bellies; take out the Guts and Gills, and if there be Roes or Livers take them out, but put them in again; flour them well, have a clear good Fire and clean Grateiron, let it be hot; lay them on, and turn them quick two or three Times for fear of sticking, and let one Side be enough; then turn the other.

This Teacher is as far out of the Art of Cookery in broiling Haddocks, as in roasting a Cod's Head: First, in putting the Roes and Livers into their Bellies; Secondly, in flouring them, and turning them quick at first on the Grateiron; for when Haddocks are in high Perfection, I will lay a Wager to broil a Haddock as soon as any Cook in *England* will broil the Roe: Then what must the Haddock be, if it is to broil till the Roe within it be enough? And

as

as for flowring and turning it fo very foon, this would cement it to the Grateirona; but if fhe would broil the Fifh whole, inftead of Flour, lay on plenty of Salt, and don't turn it till it's half broil'd, then turn it, and broil the other Side.

In Page 190, *Is to make a Scate or Thornback Soop:* Take two Pounds of Scate or Thornback, which is to be skin'd and boil'd in fix Quarts of Water; when 'tis enough take it up, pick off the Flefh and lay it by; put in the Bones again, and take two Pounds of any other Fifh, Lemon-peal, Sweet-herbs, Pepper, Mace, Horfe-raddifh, a Cruft of Bread, and Parfley, boil it to two Quarts; ftrain it off, and add an Ounce of Vermicelli, and fet it to boil; and in the mean Time take a *French* Roll, cut a little Hole in the Top, fry the Cruft brown in Batter; take the Flefh off the Fifh you laid by, and put it into a Sauce-pan, with three Spoonfuls of the Soop, Flour and Butter, Pepper and Salt; fhake them all together in a Sauce-pan till it is quite thick; then fill the Roll with it, pour your Soop into the Difh, and let the Roll fwim in the Middle.

As the Roll is filled with Fifh, fhe gives it Leave to fwim, though fhe had robb'd the Fifh, of Fins, Skin and Bones, fo that it could not fwim, neither would it let the *French* Roll fwim; therefore it muft be contented to ftand upon its own Bottom.

In Page 165, She bids, *Make a Hedge-hog thus for Change:* Two Quarts of Almonds blanched, and beat in a Mortar with Canary and Orange-flower-water, two Spoonfuls of the Tincture of Saffron, two Spoonfuls of Sorrel-juice; beat them into a fine Pafte, put in half a Pound of melted Butter, Nutmeg, Mace, Citron, and Orange, of each an Ounce, twelve Eggs, half the Whites beat up and mixed in half a Pint of Cream, a Pound of double-refined Sugar, and work it up all together; if it be not ftiff enough to make into the Form you would have it,

you

you must have a Mould for it; butter it well, then put in the Ingredients and bake it: But, says she, the Mould must be made in such a Manner as to have the Head peeping out, when it comes out of the Oven.

A Mechanical Head requires well furnished Garrets, lest the Schemes run as confused as her Way to make the Hedge-hog for Change, with such an odd Jumble as sets forth the Excellency of this Teacher's Taste and Judgment: Now, I pray, what Manner of Right hath the Tincture of Saffron, Sorrel-juice, Nutmeg, Mace, Eggs, or Cream in the Hedge-hog, baked or boiled in a Mould? If it were either reasonable that the Mould should be to make after the Hog was made; or, where can you find an Artist to make the Head peep out in the baking? Besides, she says, you may leave out the Saffron, and make it up like Chickens, or in any Shape you please; or alter the Sauce to your Fancy. Butter, Sugar, and White-wine is a pretty Sauce for either baked or boiled; or you may make the Sauce of what Colour you please; or put it into a Mould with half a Pound of Currans, and boil it for a Pudding: You may use Cocheneal instead of Saffron. She adds, Roch-allum and Cocheneal boiled in Water: This, says she, is to mix Sauces with; her Orders are to make it up like Chickens, or in any Shape you please. Now, suppose it was made in the Effigy of the Lady Teacher, garnished with Cocheneal, Roch-allum, Saffron, and Sorrel, and what other Colours the Artist fancies. She must deserve garnishing that puts Roch-allum in Sauces; for Roch-allum is an excellent Ingredient in tanning Leather for Breeches; Dyers likewise set their Colours with it; and so does the Lady Teacher set Stomachs with it.

In Page 180, To fance Eels with White-sauce: The Flesh is to be picked off the Bone of the Eel; the

Head

Head to be left whole; the Flesh is to be beat in a Mortar fine, with half the Quantity of Crumbs of Bread, Truffles, Anchovies, Pepper, Nutmeg, and Mushrooms, mix'd well with Cream with your Hand, and lay it on the Bone; but to make it in the Shape of an Eel, and bake it: For Sauce have half a Pint of Cream, and a quarter of a Pound of Butter; stir one Way till it is thick, and pour it over the Eel.

To thicken the half Pound of Butter this Teacher has ordered a Handful of Flour, and to thicken a quarter of a Pound of Butter, there is half a Pint of Cream ordered, to stir one Way till it is thick. It must not be stirred over the Fire to be made thick, for that will shortly make it thin, and the Butter will be uppermost; but in Case it is thick, where to find a Stomach that can digest Cream and a farced Eel mixed with Cream, in the above very odd Manner, I know not.

In Page 184, *Is to make a Collar of Fish in Ragoo, to look like a Breast of Veal Collar'd:* A Force-meat made of a large Eel, a Turbutt, Scate, or Thornback is to be laid on a Dresser; take away all the Bones and Fins, the Fish to be covered with the Farce; then roll it up tight, and open the Eel Skin, and bind the Collar with it nicely, so that it may be flat Top and Bottom to stand well in the Dish; then is an Earthen-dish to be buttered, upon which set the Collar upright, flour and butter it; let it be well baked, but take great Care it is not broken.

So if the Maid by her Teacher's Order takes a Turbutt, and accordingly rolls it up tight with this Eel's Skin, which must be a long one, for such a Roll will take a Skin a Yard and half long: So she sets this Collar upright in the Oven, but as soon as the Heat does pierce the Eel Skin, crack it goes; and this upright Collar may stand or fall, for the Eel Skin is no longer a Bandage for it; and instead
of

of a Collar like a roll'd Breaft of Veal, fhe may be difappointed with a broken Difh of Fifh Farce, altogether, and learn by Experience never to truft a Collar of Turbutt with an Eel Skin Bandage again.

In Page 188, is, *To Ragoo Oyfters*: This Teacher bids, take a Quart of the largeft Oyfters you can get, wafh them, fave their Liquor and make a Batter thus; take two Yolks of Eggs, grate half a Nutmeg, Lemon-peal cut fmall, a good deal of Parfley, a Spoonful of Spinage-juice, two Spoonfuls of Cream or Milk; beat all well up with Flour to a thick Batter; have ready fome Butter in a Stew-pan, and dip them one by one in the Batter; then have Crumbs of Bread, and roll them in it; fry them quick; and brown fome with the Crumbs of Bread, and fome without; then have ready a Quart of Chefnuts fheel'd, fry them, rub Butter and Flour all over the Pan; and when it is thick, then put in the Oyfter Liquor, four Blades of Mace, Piftaco Nuts fheel'd; let them boil, then put in the Chefnuts, and half a Pint of Wine; have in readinefs the Yolks of two Eggs beat up with four Spoonfuls of Cream, ftir all together; and when it is thick lay the Oyfters in the Difh, and pour the Ragoo over them.

As much as to fay, fmother the Oyfters with Hodge-podge made of Oyfter-liquor, Butter and Flour to make it thick, Yolks of Eggs and Cream to make it thicker, Chefnuts, and Piftaco Nuts, fuddled with Wine, all to fmother the Quart of large Oyfters; which upon their own Shells might appear at a Nobleman's Table, and create an Appetite; but as fhe ragoos them, creates great Trouble to the Cook, extravagant Expence to the Mafter, and deftroys Appetite: And as to her thick Batter of Cream, Eggs, Spinage-juice, and all the reft of her various Mixtures, it may be Labour in vain; although fhe dips the Oyfters in the Batter, and rolls them in Crumbs of Bread; yet ten to one but they make

make an Escape out of the Batter, and come out of the Frying a plain Oyster. If I send up Oysters in Masquerade, I put a Coat on them, and takes great Care to button it well, lest my slippery Chaps play me the Slip, and make their Escape.

In Page 201, *Is to fry Eggs as round as Balls:* Three Pints of clarified Butter is to be put into a deep Frying-pan, to be stirred with a Stick till it runs round like a Whirlpool; then is an Egg to be dropt into the Middle of it, and made as hard as potch'd Eggs; so whirl it on a Dish before the Fire: They keep hot, says she, half an Hour and be soft; so you may do as many as you please: Adds, you may serve those with what you please, but nothing better than stew'd Spinage; garnish with Orange, says she.

I say those Eggs will not be as round as Balls are, as they are to lie on a Dish half an Hour and be soft: Now had she boiled them in this Whirlpool till they had been as hard as Stones, they might have been as round as Balls; but she has but made a Dish of fry'd Eggs and Spinage: And a Dish of potched Eggs and Spinage would exceed them for Beauty, and moreover would save six Pound of Butter; for three Pints of clarified Butter will require six *London* Butter Pounds: In the next Place how far does she come short in Regard of the six Pounds of Butter to fry the twelve Eggs, concerning which she makes so much ado in her Preface, in exclaiming against the Extravagance of *French* Cooks; besides, when twelve Eggs are whirled out separately one by one, the clarified Boiling like a Whirlpool would become so black, as it would not make another Dish. Now, had this Teacher ordered the Eggs to be potched and spinaged, she would have saved the Servant a vast deal of Trouble, the Master Abundance of Butter, and me sufficient Laughing at the Whirlpool.

To make a grand Dish of Eggs: To break as many Eggs as the Yolks will fill a Pint-bason, the Whites by themselves, tie the Yolks by themselves in a Bladder round, boil them hard; then have a wooden Bowl that holds a Quart, made like two Butter-dishes, but in the Shape of an Egg, with a Hole in the Top; a String is to be run through the Bladder, and a Quarter of a Yard is to hang out at one End; this String is to be drawn through the Hole of this Dish, and then boiled; the Yolks put in, and the two Dishes clapt together and tied close, and with a fine Tunnel pour in the Whites through the Hole, which is to be stopt close, and boiled hard an Hour; then open it and cut the String close: Then put twenty Whites into two Bladders in the Shape of Eggs, boil them hard, and cut one in two Long-ways and one Cross-ways, and with a sharp Knife cut out some of the White in the Middle; the two long Halfs on each Side, with the hollow Part uppermost, and the two round flat between. Take an Ounce of Truffles and Morels, a Pint of fresh Mushrooms, a Jill of pickled Mushrooms, all chopt small: Boil sixteen of the Yolks hard and chop them; mix them with the other Ingredients, and thicken it with a Lump of Butter rolled in Flour, shaking your Pan round till it be hot and thick, says she: Then fill the two Rounds with this, turn them down again, and fill the two long ones; and what remains keep in the Sauce-pan: Add a Pint of Cream, a quarter of a Pound of Butter, the other four Yolks beat up in a Jill of White-wine, a Jill of pickled Mushrooms, Mace and Nutmeg; put all together, and stir all one Way till it is thick and fine; then pour it all over, and garnish with notched Lemon. This, says she, is a grand Dish for a second Course; or in case you should mix it with Red-wine and Butter, it will do for a first Course.

The two Butter-dishes, by my Calculation, will

H   take

take fourteen Eggs; for seven Hen Eggs I have frequently found by Experience to weigh a Pound; then are there twenty Whites hard boiled, and some of the Middle cut out: Altho' the Teacher might have made a more natural Figure, and occasioned far less Trouble, by ordering two Goose Eggs to have been hard boiled, cut Cross and Long-ways, and the Yolks would have turned out with more Ease than a Knife could cut out the Whites; and two Goose Eggs will be as big each as these ten Whites in each Bladder: Now I compute the twenty Whites of Eggs to be equal with the Bulk of ten Eggs; the Bulk of Three is cut out of the Middle of the four Halves; so there remains the Bulk of seven Eggs, which added to the other Fourteen, will make Twenty-one: To which there is for Sauce, a Quart of Mushrooms, an Ounce of Truffles and Morels, a Pint of Cream, a Jill of White-wine, sixteen Yolks of Eggs boil'd hard and cut small, which will fill a Wine-quart, of Flour, of the Yolks, the Butter boil'd in Flour, I think at least must be a Pound, whereby the Sauce will be so thick, as that a Spoon may stand in the Middle of the Sauce-pan; and withal to add more to this thick Sauce, she bids four Yolks more be beaten up; so that these twenty Yolks make this grand Dish of Eggs extravagantly abound with Mixtures: The Quart of Mushrooms might indeed have graced twenty Dishes; the Truffles and Morels ten Dishes; the Pint of Cream with part of the Yolks, helped to have made a very good Custard-pudding; the White-wine and all the Seasoning, set by for other Uses; and part of the Butter and Eggs (by Way of butter'd Eggs,) would have saved much Cost and Trouble, and made a better Dish: For the Task is hard enough for the Disher, to make out of a Quart Wooden-bowl two Butter-dishes in the Shape of an Egg, and withal to hold a Quart of Eggs. Reason is a noble Mistress

in

in Cookery; and where she does not bear Rule, how mean and contemptible does an Author appear in the Eyes of the World.

In Page 211, *Is a French Barley Pudding.* A Quart of Cream put to six Eggs well beaten, half of the Whites sweeten to your Palate, a little Orange Flower-water, a Pound of melted Butter, six Handfuls of *French* Barley, that has been boiled tender in Milk, butter a Dish and pour it in; it will take as much baking as a Venison-pasty.

But a Venison-pasty will take three Hours baking, and there is nothing in that Pudding which requires above three Quarters of an Hour baking: If the Butter be left out and three more Eggs, it will become a good Pudding; but it will be out of the Power of the tender boiled Barley and Eggs to bind the Quart of Cream and Pound of Butter together; so that there will be a Well of Oil swimming upon the Barley.

Next is, *An Apple Pudding:* To boil twelve large Pippins, after pared and cored, in four Spoonfuls of Water; and when they are soft and thick, stir in a quarter of a Pound of Butter, a Pound of Loaf-sugar, the Juice of three Lemons, the Peal of two beat in a Mortar, the Yolks of eight Eggs.

Now, my own Reason tells me, that twelve Pippins must certainly carry along with them Sharpness sufficient without the Juice of three Lemons: As also, that the bitter Peal of two Lemons will be too much bitter for twelve Pippins. I likewise aver that a Pound of Loaf-sugar is too sweet; so that this is, what I may justly call, a sour-bitter-sweet Pudding. A Spoonful Pudding is something odd; that is, a Spoonful of Flour, a Spoonful of Milk, and an Egg: Now, there should have been also a Cockle-shell to boil it in.

In the Pudding Chapter there are eleven different Puddings mentioned. In the Fast-dinner Chapter

there

there are Fifty-nine. In the Sea Captains Chapter
there are eight Puddings, in all Seventy-eight; many of them repeated three, four, five, or six Times
over, infomuch that fome of them would make one
fick of Pudding; in this F4t Chapter are eighteen
Pyes, and a Multitude of them very odd ones; one
more particular than the reft, altho' Abundance of
them exceeding miferable: I fhall however lay open
the furfeiting Quality of one, *viz. A Salt-fifh Pye:*
Take a Side of Salt-fifh, fteep and boil it, then
pick it clean from the Bones and mince it fmall;
boil a Quart of new Milk with the Crumbs of *French*
Rolls, and ftir in a Pound of Butter, and the Salt-
fifh, with Parfley, Nutmeg, Pepper, and three
Spoonfuls of Muftard; lay a good Cruft all over
your Difh, and cover it up and bake it an Hour.
Let the Reader confider whether this Salt-fifh Pye
deferves a good Cruft or no?

In Page 240, This Teacher fets out *A Chapter for
Captains of Ships to make Catchup:* Which feems
to offer Indignity to thefe brave Gentlemen,
who are the only Supports of the Nation, and
Guardians from foreign Affaults and Invafions; that
venture their Lives to bring Home rich Rubies,
Jewels, and grand Apparel to adorn Ladies with;
bringing Home all the choiceft Rarities which e-
very Nation can afford to grace their Tables with;
and all choice Wines, and rich Cordials to fupport
their Conftitutions: The Ladies might all have been
poor Cottagers, if the Sea Captains had not likewife brought Home Timber to build them their Pa-
laces. To thefe induftrious Bees, the Glory and
Ornament of the Nation, fhe orders a Gallon of ftale
Beer, Anchovies, Hot-fpices, Shalots, and two Quarts
of large Mufhroom-flaps rubbed to Pieces; which
might as well have been left out, for it would not
give the Gallon of Beer the leaft Flavour of Mufhrooms; and inftead of making good Fifh-fauce would
furfeit

furfeit the Fifh. This, fays fhe, will keep twenty
Years.

Fifh-fauce to keep the whole Year: Take twenty-four
Anchovies, ten Shalots, a Handful of fcraped Horfe-
raddifh, Mace, a Quart of White-wine, fliced Lemon, Cloves, Pepper, half a Pint of Anchovy Liquor, a Pint of Red-wine, and boil them all together
till it comes to a Quart; ftrain it off, and two
Spoonfuls will be fufficient for a Pound of Butter,
fays fhe. And further adds, it is a pretty Sauce for
boiled Fowl or Veal, or in the Room of Gravy, by
lowering it with hot Water.

A Mefs of fuch Gravy, in my Judgment, would
be a hearty Vomit.

This Lady gives a Receipt to *Pot Dripping:* Take,
fays fhe, fix Pounds of Beef-dripping; boil it eight
Times; all the Gravy on the In-fide muft be fcraped
off; then is it to be tinctured with Bay-leaves, Cloves,
Pepper, Salt, and ftrained thro' a Sieve into a Pot,
when quite cold, cover it up: Thus, fays fhe, you
may do what Quantity you pleafe. And the beft
Way to keep any Sort of Dripping is to turn the
Pot upfide down, and then the Rats cannot get at
it. She fays, if it will keep on Ship-board, it will
make as fine Puff-pafte Cruft, as any Butter can do,
or Cruft for Puddings.

But, I fay, the Difference betwixt Dripping Puff-
pafte and Butter Puff-pafte, is as difproportionate as
Pebbles are from Diamonds: Befides, I can never a-
gree in Opinion with the Lady Teacher, for the
Drippings to be fhipped off, and that for two Reafons: Firft, I don't think it reafonable that thefe
brave Heroes fhould be fed with Kitchen-ftuff Pyes
or Puddings: Cruft made of Dripping muft lie hea-
vy upon the Stomachs of thefe brave Men, and cannot but difturb their active Souls. My fecond Reafon is, that the Kitchen Of-falls are given to fupport the Poor by charitable Gentry; and are the
Cooks

Cooks Perquifites in Noblemens Families, which are
purchafed by the Poor at a cheaper Rate than Butter: With them Dripping may be a delicious Morfel to fupport Hunger; but what Lady before this
Teacher ever found out fuch Virtue in Beef-drippings? I know not, for the Chance which they
have of catching Cinders and Afhes would (I fhould
think) fet the Ladies Stomachs againft it: Yet,
fuch is the Delicacy of this Lady Teacher, as that
in her Orders to bake Fifh, fhe bids, lay it in a
Difh and ftick fome Bits of Butter, or fine Dripping on the Fifh. And in Pea-foop, fhe orders falt
Pork to be boiled in it. Likewife, orders for a
Pudding, that a good Cruft be made with Dripping; and five Pounds of falt Pork to boil four
or five Hours in this good Dripping Cruft. Nay,
fix Puddings more fhe has ordered, and not fo much
as one Egg amongft them all.

In Page 251, *Is to pot Pigeons or Fowls:* This
Teacher bids feafon them pretty well with Pepper
and Salt, and bake them in Butter till they are tender; then drain them from the Gravy, lay them in
a Cloth that will fuck all the Gravy up, and feafon
them again with Salt and Pepper, Mace and Cloves:
They are to be put down clofe in a Pot, and cover'd
with Butter near an Inch thick above the Birds:
Thus, fays fhe, you may do all Sorts of Fowl, only
wild Fowl fhould be boned.

To feafon potted Fowl with fo much hot Spices,
and to prefs out the Juice or Gravy, fets forth the
Teacher's Judgment in cold as well as hot Difhes;
for next fhe pots a cold Tongue, beats it in a Mortar with melted Butter and two Anchovies till its mel-
low; then puts it in Pots and covers it with clarified
Butter: Thus, fays fhe, you may do wild Fowl.

How various and changeable is this Lady, when
fhe orders fo much hot Spices above! but here fays
not one Word of it: Two Anchovies chopt in cold

Tongue

Tongue or wild Fowl, would surfeit both : Can any
Thing eat better than a well cured Tongue? or did
any ever beat wild Fowl with Anchovies to pot ? But
she tells a second and third Way to pot Tongues,
and to pot Beef like Venison; namely, for eight
Pounds of Beef she takes four Ounces of Salt-petre,
four Ounces of Peter-salt, a Pint of coarse Salt, an
Ounce of Sal-prunella; the Beef is to be cut into
pound Pieces and rubb'd with these Salts, to lie four
Days, turning them every Day, and bake them tender as a Chicken; drain the Gravy from them, take
out all the Skins and Sinews; pound it in a Morter,
and mix it with an Ounce of Cloves and Mace, three
quarters of an Ounce of Pepper, and a Nutmeg, all
beat very fine; mix all well with the Meat, put clarified Butter to moisten it, and lay it down in Pots very hard; set it at the Oven Mouth just to settle, says she.

Indeed, so very great a Heat she has given it with
Salts and hot Seasonings, might require such a set-
tling as it would not get in the Oven's Mouth; and,
says she, cover it two Inches thick with clarified
Butter : To this add eight Pounds of Beef, (there
are Salts sufficient to colour a whole Beef red) and
when it is baked tender, all the Sinews and Skin
taken out, there will not be five Pounds; to which
she puts an Ounce of Cloves and Mace; a Quantity
which I would not put in five Stone of potted Beef,
and would make it eat more like Venison than she
has done.

Next, *Page* 254, she pots *Cheshire Cheese:* She
pounds three Pounds of *Cheshire* Cheese with half a
Pound of Sweet-butter, half a Pint of fine Canary,
and half an Ounce of Mace beat and sifted like
a fine Powder; and when all is extremely well mixed, press it hard down into a Gally-pot and set it
in a cool Place, after covering it with clarified Butter; a Slice of this, she says, exceeds all the Cream
Cheese that can be made: If she would have but
told

told the Truth, she should have added, is invented for a Surfeit.

Now, I think, there are few Persons who are acquainted with Cream Cheese, but like it wondrous well; but then was ever powder'd Mace put into it? And if it be old *Cheshire* with the Mace, it would take the Skin off one's Mouth: Was ever such a Mixture in Cheese recommended by a Lady to exceed Cream Cheese, which is so mild that not one Grain of Salt is to be put into it, if it be right made? So there is Ten-pence for Mace, to powder; Nine-pence for a Jill of rich Canary; half a Pound of Butter to beat into the Mixture, and a Pound to clarify, in order to cover this Surfeit of potted *Cheshire* Cheese.

Next, she *Collars a Breast of Veal or a Pig:* And amongst the rest of her Ingredients, bids, Penny-royal to be put in.

Next again, *Is to Collar Beef:* She bids take a thin Piece of flank Beef, and slip the Skin to the End, and dissolve a Quart of Petre-salt; after beating the Beef with a Rolling-pin, it is to be put into five Quarts of Pump-water, and to lie five Days; plenty of hot Spices is to be laid on the Beef, and the Skin is to be laid on again, to roll it tight; put it in a Pot, with a Pint of Claret, and to bake it in the Oven with Bread.

In the first Place, the thin Piece of flank Beef is a small Piece for such a large Quantity of Petre-salt, sufficient to colour two Bacon Hogs; and what Reason can she shew for stripping the Skin to the End of the Beef, and to bid bake it, and tell us no more about it: For colour'd Beef is not finished when baked.

So she prescribes another Way to season a Collar of Beef; to which she doubles the Quantity of hot Spices, and adds a quarter of an Ounce of Coriander-seeds; a sufficient Quantity to fuddle a hundred

Dares

Dares; then bakes it in the Pickle, and hangs it in
a Net three Days within the Air of the Fire; then
puts it in a clean Cloth, and hangs it within the Air
of the Fire. A new and very odd Manner of collaring Beef.

In Page 204, is a Farce Meagre Cabbage: This
Teacher bids take a white Heart Cabbage, as big
as the Bottom of a Plate, and to boil just five Minutes in Water; then to take out the Inside, leaving
the outside Leaves whole; chop what you take
out very fine, with the Fish of three Flounders clean
pick'd from the Bone, four hard Eggs, a Handful
of Parsley, chop all well together; mixt up with
the Yolk of an Egg, a few Crumbs of Bread, and
a quarter of a Pound of Butter; all to be stuff'd into
the Cabbage, and tye it together; put it into a deep
Stew-pan, with half a Pint of Water, a quarter of
a Pound of Butter rolled in Flour, the Yolks of
four hard Eggs, Onion, Cloves, white Pepper, Mace,
half an Ounce of Truffles and Morels, Catchup, and
pickled Mushrooms; cover it close and let it simmer
an Hour; if it is not enough you must do it longer:
Untye and lay it on a Dish, and pour the Sauce
over, says she.

I agree with this Lady, that the white Cabbage
is the poorest of all Cabbages, that is the Product of
any Herd's Garth, and the real Value cannot be a-
bove a Half-penny; to which there is half a Pound
of Butter Four-pence, Eggs Three-pence, Flounders
Three-pence, Truffles and Morels Nine-pence, hot
Spices, Catchup and Mushrooms, I call Six-pence;
which in all amounts to two Shillings and a Penny,
to farce and sauce this Half-penny Cabbage; and when
it is done, if Man, Woman or Child, Hog, Sow or
Dog eat it, my Judgment deceives me.

In Page 225, Is a Salt-fish Pye: She bids boil a
Side of Salt-fish tender, and let it be minced small;
then take the Crumbs of two *French* Rolls cut in

I   Slices,

Slices, boil up with a Quart of new Milk, and put
to it your minced Salt-fish, a Pound of melted Butter, two Spoonfuls of minced Parſley, half a Nutmeg, beaten Pepper, three Spoonfuls of Muſtard;
mix all well together; make a good Cruſt and lay
all over your Diſh, and cover it up; then bake it an
Hour.

Will any reaſonable Perſon ſay, this Salt-fiſh Pye
deſerves a good Cruſt? And if Remedies were not
more dangerous than Diſeaſes, why may not old
left-off Shoes come in Vogue and Uſe.

In Page 258, this Teacher ſets forth *How to make
Pork Hams:* To a Ham of fat Pork is a Pound of
coarſe Sugar, a Pound of common Salt, an Ounce
of Salt-petre mixt together; and the Ham to be laid
in a wooden Tray, bathing it every Day with the
Pickle, in which the Ham is to lie one Month; then
to be hung up in Wood Smoak, and after put into
a damp Place a Month or two to make it mouldy,
that it may cut ſhort and fine: And never lay theſe
Hams in Water till you boil them, which muſt be
in a Copper or the biggeſt Pot you have; put it in
cold Water, and let it be four Hours before it boils;
skim it well and often till it boils: If it be a large
one, two Hours will boil it. Take it up half an
Hour before Dinner, skin it and throw Raſpings over
it: She adds, after all to be ſure to boil the Ham
in as much Water as you can, and to keep it skim-
ing all the Time it boils.

A very particular Way of the Teacher's curing
Ham, as well as boiling it. For eight Pounds of
Beef for Potting, ſhe orders nine Ounces of Salts;
and to 20 Pounds of Pork, (for that will be the
Weight of a good Ham) ſhe orders one Ounce of
Salts, a Pound of Sugar, and a Pound of Salt well
mixt, and rubb'd on the Ham; then laid in a hol-
low Tray for the Pickle to ſwell about it, and to
baſte it every Day (with its own Liquor) for one
Month.

Month. Now, suppose that the whole national Product of Hams in one Year, could be cured by this Teacher's Orders, *viz.* with an equal Quantity of Sugar and Salt. In the first Place, the Teacher's Extravagancy would be obvious to any, though of never so weak a Capacity, the Price of Sugar and Salt compar'd: Secondly, What would still be of worse Consequence, would be the Loss of all the Hams; for the Sugar would sweeten the Salt so much, as to entirely disable it from penetrating into the Bones of them; therefore consequently must putrify, when put into Trays, Troughs, or Tubs a Month, and all the Liquor to swell about them; the Spirits of which co-operating with the Juices of the Hams, would work like a Gile-fat, and in a Month's Time stink worse than any Carrion. *Yorkshire*, says she, is famous for Hams; and the Reason is, that their Salt is much finer than ours in *London*; it being a large clear Salt, and gives the Meat a fine Flavour. And further informs you, that she used to have it from *Malden* in *Essex*; and that, the very same Salt (*viz.* of *Malden*) will make any Ham as fine as you can desire. How strangely ungrateful is *Yorkshire* with its famous Salt, in furnishing *Malden* in *Essex* therewith, and letting the greatest Metropolis of the Kingdom want so necessary a Seasoning: So that this Teacher could not get proper Salt for her Hams, except she got it from *Malden*; and by the Strength of such Salt, and herself-sufficiency, by setting forth its Virtues so largely and clearly, which if it should exceed Glass itself, the Method she takes to use it would both destroy its Virtue and Beauty. The Lady further recommends, that Tongues put into the above Pickle, and to lie for a Fortnight, they will be fine either immediately boil'd, or Wood smoked.

In her 16th *Page*, she informs you, *How to keep Hares or Venison sweet, and make them fresh, if they stink.*

In

In *Page* 259, fhe fays, that fhe has feen *potted Birds* fo bad, as that no Perfon could bear the Smell thereof; and that by managing of them, fhe has made them as good as ever were cat.

The former fhe made fweet, firft, by wafhing in warm Water; fecondly, in Luke-warm Milk and Water; then by drying, and rubbing them all over with Ginger, and hanging them in an airy Place: The latter fhe made good by lying half a Minute in boiling Water; then applying Pepper, Salt, and Mace to them; fcald their Pot, and cover with frefh Butter. I think the Teacher fhews the ignorant Servant the Way to make Hams and Tongues ftink, but gives no Directions how to make them frefh, except it be by fkimming the Ham fix Hours: And if a Ham require that Time, how many Cooks and Slaves would an elegant Entertainment require? Now, my own private Judgment gives me to underftand, that fix Hours fkimming a Ham will in no Cafe avail to fweeten a bad one, but may be of Service to the Broth, by taking off the grofs Fat, which might make the Hogs fick: And I muft own, if the Hogs could fhew any Gratitude to their Benefactrefs, they are under a far greater Obligation to the Lady, than Gentry are for her *Portable Soop* eight or nine Hours boil'd without fkimming. Such monftrous prodigious Inconfiftences I am afham'd any Cook fhould recommend, efpecially a Lady; and had I not her Inftructions lying before me, I muft acknowledge I fhould have been like St. *Thomas*, for his Unbelief. But finding her Treatife hugely abounding with fuch Inconfiftencies and naufeous Inftructions, I fhall not give my Readers any further Trouble with them in my Book,

PRO.

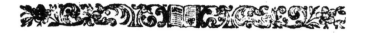

PROFESSED
COOKERY.

A White Fricassey of Chickens.

TAKE four Chickens and skin them, take out their Back-bones and cut them into Joints, leaving their Breasts whole; wash them very clean, and melt a Pound and a Half of sweet Butter in a small Hash-pan, on a very slow Stove, into which put your Chickens; add to them three Blades of Mace, six Cloves, half a Nutmeg bruised, and let them simmer an Hour and an Half, but not boil: In which Time wash clean the Back-bones, Necks and Gizzards of them. Add to them a Quart of Water, and put them into a Sauce-pan covered close; let them stew till they come to half a Pint, then strain it off; and when the Fricassey is tender, pour out the Butter and take out the Chickens: Clean the Pan, and skim the Butter clean from the Gravy, and strain it into the Hash-pan, into which put your Fricassey; add to it the half Pint of Gravy, and set it on a Stove; boil six Eggs hard and take out the Yolks; then take a Jill of thick Cream, and add to it some Butter and Flour, and put them into the Fricassey; and when it boils, toss it up, and squeeze in the Juice of a Lemon, and set the Breasts with their Points square in the Middle of the Dish, and lay the Joints round the Yolks of
Eggs,

Eggs, and broiled Livers all over, and pour on your
Sauce: Then lay green Parſley and carved Lemon
round the Diſh, and ſtrew a little cut Parſley over
the Fricaſſey, and ſend it up.

Another *White Fricaſſey of* Chickens.

TAKE three well grown Chickens, blood them
and pick off their Feathers, skin and cut them
in Joints, and beat their Breaſts flat; waſh them
clean in warm Water, and lay them in a Stew-pan,
and put thereto as much ſoft Water as will cover
them, a Blade of Mace and half a Nutmeg ſliced:
Let them ſtew on a ſlow Stove till they are tender;
then take them out of the Broth they are ſtew'd in,
let it boil to half a Pint, and ſtrain it through a
clean Hair-ſieve; waſh clean the Pan, into which
put the Gravy, add half a Pint of Cream; or if you
have not Cream, take the Quantity of Milk, adding
double the Quantity of very ſweet Butter, which
makes it as rich as the Cream: Toſs it up after it is
boil'd, thicken it with the Juice of a Lemon and a
Spoonful of pickled Muſhrooms: Lay Sippets and
Parſley round the Diſh, and ſerve it up.

To make a *White Fricaſſey of* Rabbets.

TAKE young Rabbets and skin them, waſh the
Blood clean from them, dry them well with a
clean coarſe Towel, and cut them in Joints; ſeaſon
them with Mace and Nutmeg, and take a quarter of
a Pound of Butter into a clean Frying-pan, ſet it on
a very ſlow Stove, and keep it turning all the Time
it is frying that it may not Brown; and when it is
tender pour off the Butter; add half a Jill of Cream,
white Veal-gravy the ſame Quantity, put thereto
three Spoonfuls of thick melted Butter, boil'd Truffles and Morels very tender in Gravy, and make a
Border of them round the Fricaſſey; the two Rabbets Heads in the Middle, with their Jaw-bones ſtuck
into

into their [ ]. Lay sippets round the Dish, with Parsley
and [ ]-berries for Garnish.

Another White Fricassey of Rabbets

WHEN you cannot get young Rabbets, and muſt
have a White Fricaſſey, old Rabbets have a
ſtrong Taſte, which may be corrected by taking half
a Jill of Verjuice, and after you have waſhed and
cut the Rabbets into little Pieces, turn every one of
theſe Pieces over in the Verjuice, and add a Pint of
Water; take Care that the Water be ſoft, for hard
Water will turn them red: Let them boil ſoftly in
this Water and Verjuice ten Minutes; then pour it
all out, and add to them a Pint of White-gravy;
let there be a Tea Spoonful of White-pepper and
three Blades of Mace tied in a Muſlin-rag, and boil
on a very ſlow Stove till the Rabbets are tender, by
which Time the better Half of the Gravy will be
conſum'd; then take out your Spices, add to the
Fricaſſey a Jill of Cream, and about half a Jill of
Muſhrooms: Thicken your Sauce with a little Flour
wrought up in Butter, viz. lay half a Spoonful of
Flour on a Plate, take a Piece of Butter, and with
the Back of a Spoon work up the Flour into the
Butter; and when you put it into the Fricaſſey, toſs
it up all the Time the Butter is diſſolving: So lay
Sippets and Parſley round your Diſh, and ſerve it
up.

A Brown Fricaſſey of Rabbets.

SKIN the Rabbets, but keep the Ears on their
Heads, and rub them over with Butter, after
that the Yolk of an Egg; then grate ſome Bread
and rub over the Heads; pin the Ears upon white
Paper at their full Length, or roaſt them in a Dripping-pan, or ſet them in an Oven; then cut the
Rabbets into little Pieces, ſave the three hind Parts,
and

and let their Tails be rubb'd with [ ] grated bread; broil and baste them with melted butter: Then season the Fricassey with Mace, Pepper, Nutmeg; flour and fry them a fine light brown; then take a Quart of brown Gravy into a Stew-pan, put in your Fricaſſey, and let it boil on a flow Stove till there is juſt Gravy ſufficient for Sauce: To which add Force-meat Balls, a Spoonful of Walnut-pickle or Catchup; ſlice two or three ſmall Girkins, and add to it: Then toſs up your Fricaſſey with a little of thick melted Butter; lay Sippets round the Diſh; ſet the hind Parts of the Rabbets with the Tails on the Middle of the Fricaſſey; take off the Papers from the Ears; and take out the Jaw-bones and put into their Eyes; then ſet them round the Fricaſſey. This ſerves for a Top-diſh, in a firſt and ſecond Courſe.

A Brown Fricaſſey of Chickens.

TAKE four Chickens, skin and cut them into Joints, only leave the Breaſt-bones whole, flat them with a Bill-knife, and ſeaſon them with Nutmeg, Pepper, and Salt; flour and fry them Brown: Seaſon all the Livers of the Chickens, dip them in Yolks of Eggs, and grate Bread over them; broil them before the Fire on a Tin-pan, baſte them well with Butter, and turn them till they are criſp; then put them into a Stew-pan, with a Jill of ſtrong brown Gravy; add pickled Muſhrooms, Catchup, ſome Aſparagus-tops boil'd tender in hard Water, cut in Lengths and Breadth of your Thumb: Add them to the Gravy, with a Tea Cupful of plain melted Butter: Then put in your Fricaſſey, and toſs it up on a clear Stove or Fire till it boils; and lay it on a Diſh with the four Breaſts uppermoſt, the Livers to be laid round the Fricaſſey. Garniſh with ſliced Lemon, and green pickled Girkin.

A

A White Fricassey of Veal

TAKE a [   ] of a leg of veal and stuff it
with force-meat, sew it up, and boil it
with half a Pound of Veal put into a Sauce-pan,
a Quart of Water, two Shalots, some White-
pepper, and two Blades of Mace; slice half a Nutmeg, which add to it: Let it boil gently till there
be three Jills consumed; then cut out of the Leg
of Veal a thick Piece, about the Breadth of two of
your Fingers, and the Length of one; cut it thin,
and season it very lightly with Nutmeg and Salt;
then beat the Whites of two Eggs very well, and
dip the Veal into the Eggs, flour it, and have some
clarified Butter in a Frying-pan, with a clear Fire;
and when the Butter is hot, be very quick and lay
in the Veal: One Minute will do it. It must be
crisp and white; take Care not to lose one Drop of
its Gravy. And when you have fry'd all the Veal,
cover it and keep it hot before the Fire; strain off
the Gravy, skim it well, take out the Udder, rub
it over with the Yolk of an Egg, grate Bread over
it, and crisp it before the Fire, cut some Parsley
small, and throw over it; then take the Gravy and
half a Jill of thick Cream, a Piece of Butter wrought
up in Flour, put them into a Sauce-pan, and toss it
up; and when it is smooth, squeeze in half a Lemon, or a Spoonful of Verjuice; then lay your Veal
round the Dish, pour on the Sauce, set the Udder in
the Middle: Garnish with Parsley and green Pickles.

A Yellow Fricassey of Chickens.

TAKE three Chickens; pick and singe them
well, cut them up their Backs, wash all the
Blood from their Bones, flat them with the Side of
a Bill-knife; then season them with Mace and Salt,
and fry them on a slow Stove a Quarter of an Hour:
Then add to them a Quart of fair Water, and let
them

them ſtew till they are tender, and rill ſuch Time as there's juſt as much Liquor as is ſufficient for the Sauce: Then take a Pennyworth of Saffron, infuſe it into a Glaſs of Rheniſh-wine, and broil the Chicken Livers; add to them half a Jill of Muſhrooms: And after you have extracted all the Colour from the Saffron, ſtrain the Wine into the Fricaſſey; thicken it with Butter and Flour, toſs it up; lay the Chickens whole on the Diſh, and pour the Sauce over them; lay the broiled Livers round them: Garniſh with Parſley and carved Lemon.

A *Red Fricaſſey of* Chickens.

DO the Chickens as above directed; adding to them the ſame Quantity of Water; take ſome red Berries of a Lobſter, bruiſe and boil them in a Jill of Water, and ſtrain them through a Hair-ſieve into the Fricaſſey; add to it ſome Force-meat Balls: And when it is ſtewed to a Gravy ſufficient for Sauce, thicken it with a little drawn Butter; and broil the Livers and Gizzards, and lay them round the Fricaſſey: Garniſh as above directed.

A *Green Fricaſſey of* Chickens.

SINGE, ſeaſon and fry three Chickens as above directed; boil an hundred of the Tops of Aſparagus in Water, and add to the Chickens; then melt a Quarter of a Pound of Butter; make it very Green with Sorrel beaten in a Mortar, and the Juice ſtrained into the Butter; boil Parſley, and mix it with the Butter: Then when the Chickens are ſtewed till there is left about juſt half a Pint of Liquor, toſs in the green Butter and Parſley: Toſs it up, lay your Chickens in the Diſh, with the Aſparagus-tops round them, pour over the green Sauce: Garniſh with Parſley, and ſerve it up.

N. B. By theſe above-mentioned Receipts, you may fricaſſey Partridge, Pigeons, Lamb or Veal.

To

To ragoo a Breast of Veal.

TAKE the thick Brisket-part of the Breast of Veal; cut it in thick Slices, and set it on to stove in a Stew-pan; add to it two Quarts of Water and cover it close: Then bone the thin Part of it, and make a savoury Force-meat, and rub the Inside of the Veal with the Yolk of an Egg; upon which lay a thin Lair of Force-meat: Then roll up the Veal tight, and put it into a Pot, and let it stand two Hours in an Oven; the other stewing all the Time over a slow Stove: Add to it two Veal Sweet-breads cut in Pieces, Truffles and Morels: Boil two Beef-palates tender, and cut into Dices, some pickled Mushrooms; and when the Gravy is consumed to a Quantity sufficient for Sauce, thicken it up, and pour it into a Dish; set the Roll in the Middle: Garnish the Dish with Lemon.

To make Scotch Collops.

TWO Pounds of Veal will make a middling Dish of Collops. Cut them very thin and season them with Mace, Nutmeg and Pepper, and fry them of a light Brown; and as you fry them, cover them close up, and set them before the Fire: Put into the Frying-pan a little strong Broth, boil it and pour into a Porringer; so rub out your Pan exceeding clean: Put in more Butter and fry all the Collops; and put them to the other Collops: Then take Gravy into the Frying-pan and boil it up, and strain it through a clean Sieve into a Sauce-pan; take twenty Force-meat Balls and fry them; add to the Sauce a Spoonful of Catchup, two Artichoke-bottoms cut in Quarters; boil up your Sauce: Dish up your Collops, pour on your Sauce, and lay over your fryed Balls with Rashers of Bacon, and so serve it up.

Stuffed

Stuffed Scotch Collops.

CUT your Collops out of the thick Part of the
Leg of Veal; let them be thin, and rub every
Collop with the Yolk of an Egg: Then, have ready
ſome ſavoury Fonce-meat, and ſpread a thin Lair
over every Collop, and lay it double; cut it ſquare,
and lay them on a flat-bottomed Earthen-diſh well
buttered; upon which ſtrow over grated Bread:
Then ſet them in an Oven of an equal Heat Top
and Bottom, till they are of a light Brown. In the
mean Time take the Fragments you cut off the Collops, and fry them Brown; add two Pints of Water,
two Shalots, an Anchovy, Jamaica and Black-pepper; and let it boil gently till three Jills be conſum'd: Then ſtrain it, and add thereto a Spoonful
of Muſhrooms; take a Sauce-pan and a little Butter,
boil it up, and pour it over the Diſh, upon which
lay your Stuff Collops: Garniſh with green Pickles.

To make larded Scotch Collops.

TAKE a Fillet-piece of a Leg of Veal, and cut
five large Collops off it; lard them all over
with very clear and well cured Bacon, and cut ſome
Collops very thin; beat and ſeaſon them with Nutmeg, Mace, Pepper and Salt: Seaſon the larded
Collops on the Under-ſide, which is not the Side
that is larded; fry them in clarified Butter, and after
them the other Collops. Then have ready ſome
ſtrong brown Gravy, Catchup a Spoonful, ſome
Muſhrooms, or Truffles and Morels boiled tender in
Water, and after in the Gravy: Fry Force-meat Balls,
and put the plain Collops into a Haſh-pan, where
the Gravy and other Ingredients are, and toſs them
up over a clear Stove or Fire: Diſh them up, and
lay four of the larded Collops round the Bottom,
and on the Middle: Garniſh with carved Lemon and
ſliced Cucumber.

Veal

Veal in Blankets

Cut out of a Fillet of Veal six Collops which must be five inches long, and four broad; beat and season them with Nutmeg, Pepper and Salt; rub them all over with the Yolk of an Egg, then take Savoury-meat and lay on every Collop a thin Lair; make some cold Paste of a Quart of Flour, into which rub six Ounces of Butter very small a-mongst the Flour; beat up an Egg with as much Water as will make a stiff Paste; then cut it into six sheets, and roll them into squares, something larger than your Collops: Roll up your Collops, after that roll them in this Paste, every one must be roll'd in a clean Cloth, and to be boil'd an Hour: Then take them up, set three in the Dish with their Ends in the Middle, cut the other three down the Middle, lay the Cut-side uppermost, and two Cut-halfs between each whole one: For Sauce, Gravy and Butter, send it up hot.

To Make Veal Olives

TAKE four Collops of the same Bigness as a-bove-taught, and lay Yolks of Eggs, Seasoning and Force-meat, in the aforesaid Manner; then cut out of the Belly-part of Bacon eight Rashers, every Rasher so long as to lap round the rolled Veal, two rashers to ever Roll; lay them on a flat-bot-tom'd Earthen-plate, and set them in an oven three Quarters of an Hour: Then have ready half a Jill of good Gravy, take out your Veal Olives, and pour out the Fat from them; lay them on the Dish, and the Gravy that they discharg'd in the Oven; pour in the other Gravy: Boil it up, and pour into the other Dish wherein the Olives are, and so serve it up.

A Breaſt of Veal *Ragoo'd.*

TAKE a Breaſt of Veal, bone and cut it with a ſharp Knife on the Upper-ſide, by way of checker Work a-croſs; make of Bacon and Lemon-skin Lardens an Inch long, and lard the Breaſt all over the Upper-ſide with them of each an equal Quantity, by Way of Mixture: Turn the other Side and ſeaſon it with Nutmeg, Pepper and Salt; half roaſt it before the Fire; then have ready a Quart of Gravy in a large Stew-pan over a ſlow Stove, into which put your Breaſt of Veal, cover the Pan cloſe: Then take an Ox-foot, and cut the cloven Part betwixt the Hoofs into very ſmall Dices, by Way of Ox-palates; it is exceeding fine, and anſwers to the ſame Purpoſe: Take 20 Force-meat Balls fry'd, and when your Liquor is half waſted, add the Balls and Ox-foot; when you find the Veal very tender, have ready two Sweet-breads brown broiled, cut them in Dices, and add to the Ragoo: And when the Gravy is conſumed to ſuch a Quan-as is juſt ſufficient for Sauce, take 20 freſh Oyſters bearded, and put them into the Ragoo a Minute before you ſend it up: Lay Sippers and carved Lemon round the Diſh; then lay on the Veal, and pour over the Ragoo.

To ragoo a Fillet of Veal.

CUT a Fillet of Veal, ſtuff it with ſavoury Force-meat, and put it into an Earthen-pot with half a Pint of Water; cover it over with two Sheets of Cap-paper, and tye it with Pack-thread; ſet it in an Oven three Hours: In which Time take a Pound of Beef, cut it into thin Slices, and take a Slice of Butter into a Stew-pan, and fry the Beef brown: Then put in three Pints of Water, two Shalots, and an Anchovy; let it boil very gently till one Pint

is

is conſumed, then ſtrain it off into a Sauce-pan:
Add to it half an Ounce of Truffles and Morels, and
let them boil tender; likewiſe two Artichoke-bottoms cut in Quarters, Force-meat Balls, an Ox-palate
boiled tender and cut in Pieces; add to this the
Ragoo. And when the Veal is enough, take it out
of the Oven, pour off the Gravy from it, skim off
the Fat, and ſtrain the Gravy into the Ragoo: Then
lay the Fillet of Veal on a Diſh, pour over it the
Ragoo, and lay Sippets round the Diſh and carved
Lemon.

A Pokey Tongue.

TAKE a large Loin of Lamb, make Force-meat
of the Kidney and Fat; take out the Chine-
bone, cut all the Lean in Slices, and lay them in
the Form of a boiled Tongue, a Lair of Force-meat
and one of Lamb: When you have made it in the
Form of a Beef's Tongue, cover it all over with
Force-meat; ſet it in an Oven an Hour and a Half:
For Sauce, have ſome brown Gravy and Capers:
Set the Tongue on the Diſh, and ſerve it up.

A Pallateen.

CUT out of the thick Part of a Leg of Veal
a Pound and a Half into round Slices; take
three Quarters of a Pound of ſavoury Force-meat,
and ſeaſon the Veal with Salt, Pepper, and Nutmeg;
lay the Kell of the Veal in the Bottom of a round
Pot: Then lay a Slice of Veal upon the Kell, and
upon the Veal a Lair of Force-meat; ſo Veal upon that, till all is laid in Lairs: Set it in an Oven
an Hour and a Half; and for Sauce take the Gravy
that it diſcharges, skimming off all the Fat: Add to
it a Spoonful of Catchup, the Juice of half a Lemon; likewiſe half a Jill of good Gravy, thickened
with a little melted Butter: Set the Pallateen in the
Diſh;

Diſh; and ſlice Girkin or pickle Cucumber, for garniſhing: Then ſerve it up.

A Calf's Head *Haſh.*

BE very careful of taking the Brains whole out of the Head; let it be very well waſhed, and boiled in ſoft Water: Take a Pound of Veal and cut it in thin Slices, fry it in a Stew-pan with Butter till it is brown; then take three Pints of the Broth that it was boiled in, and put into the Pan to the fry'd Veal; add to it Sweet-marjoram and Thyme: Let all boil till it is good; then cut One-half of the Head into thin Slices, ſtrain off the Gravy from the Veal and Herbs; ſeaſon the Head with Mace, Nutmeg, and Pepper; put it into the Haſh-pan with the Gravy, and let it ſtew over a ſlow Stove: Then take the other Half of the Head, and cut off the Scull-bone and Mouth: Cut it with a ſharp Knife a-croſs, and rub it with the Yolk of an Egg; grate Bread over, and brown it before the Fire, baiting it with Butter, and ſtrew over it ſome green Parſley cut ſmall: Then take the Brains, and take off the red Strings they are covered with, dip them in Egg, ſtrew over them ſome grated Bread, and have ſome boiling Fat to fry the Brains in; add 20 Forcemeat Balls, half a Jill of pickled Muſhrooms: And when the Haſh is very tender, and there is no more Gravy than is proper for Sauce to it, pour in a little melted Butter: Lay carved Sippets round the Diſh, and pour on your Haſh. Set the broiled Half in the Middle, with Raſhers of Bacon over it, and the fry'd Brains on each Side.

To haſh a Calf's Head *White.*

BOIL the Calf's Head in the above Manner, take out the Brains as aforeſaid, and take two Quarts of the Liquor that the Head was boiled in: Add to
it

it a Pound of Veal cut into little Pieces, two Blades
of Mace, a Nutmeg cut into Slices, an Onion, and
a little White-pepper; cut the one Side of the Head
in Slices; and when the White-gravy is confumed
to one Quart, ſtrain it off, waſh your Haſh-pan,
and put in the Haſh and Gravy, and let it ſtew till
the Gravy is half confumed; then make twenty
Balls of white Force-meat and put into the Haſh
unfry'd: Add a Spoonful of Muſhrooms; dip the
Brains in Eggs and fry them: Add to the Haſh
half a Jill of thick Cream. Garniſh the Diſh with
Sippets and green Parſley; toſs up your Haſh and
pour it into the Diſh: Lay the Brains in the Middle, and ſome Raſhers of Bacon round.

How to ſtew the other Side of the Head.

CUT a Pound of Veal or Beef thin, and fry it
brown with Butter: Add to it two Quarts of
the Broth the Head was boiled in: Add to it likewiſe a Rocombal, this is a Sort of Garlick that is
red, and exceeds Shalot or Onion; then take ſix
Lamb-ſtones, and ſix Suckles, fry them brown, but
ſeaſon them with Nutmeg, Pepper and Salt firſt,
and cut every Lamb-ſtone in two; then ſtrain off
the Gravy clean out of the Pan, and put in the half
Head, Lamb-ſtones, and Suckles: Add ſome pickled
Kidney-beans cut ſmall; thicken the Gravy with Butter and Flour: Lay the half Head in the Middle,
the Stones and Suckles round it fry'd: Parſley and
green Pickles for garniſhing.

To ſtew a Lamb's Head *and* Pluck.

TAKE a Lamb's Head, take the Skin off it, and
take out the Eyes, cut the Liver in two; waſh
the Head and Pluck very clean, and put it into a
large Sauce-pan to boil; take half of the Liver,
and beat it in a Marble Mortar, or ſhred it on a
Board,

Board, grate ſome Bread, Thyme, Sweet-marjoram,
Parſley, Nutmeg, Pepper, Salt, an Egg, and a Slice
of ſweet Butter, work it up with your Hand, and
put it into a Piece of clean Linen Cloth, and boil
it with the Head and Pluck; then cut the other
half of the Liver very thin, and fry it in a Haſh-pan
with Butter and two Raſhers of Bacon Ham; then
take the Broth the Lamb's Head and Pluck were
boiled in, and pour it into the Haſh-pan and let it
boil; boil thirty Aſparagus, cut off their Tops, and
add them to the Haſh; then pour in a little melted
Butter, and take the boiled forced Liver cut into
Slices; then pour the Haſh into the Diſh: Set the
Head in the Middle, lay over the Head and Haſh
the ſliced forced Liver, and ſerve it up.

How to dreſs a Veal's Pluck.

TAKE one of the beſt Veal's Pluck you can get,
take off the Liver, Heart, and Cat's-collop;
and ſet on the Lights to boil in a large Sauce-pan
that has a Cover; put Water to it, cover it cloſe,
and ſet it on the Fire to boil; then take half a Pound
of the Veal's Liver, a quarter of a Pound of Beef-
ſuet ſhred ſmall with the Liver; ſeaſon it with Parſley, Thyme, Sweet-marjoram, Nutmeg, Pepper and
Salt: Add to it one Egg, and a little grated Bread,
tie this in a Piece of clean Linen, and boil it with
the Lights: Add to it Shalots, and Sweet-herbs;
then cut the Veal's Heart into thin Slices, and fry
in a Haſh-pan with Butter; cut three Slices of the
Liver and fry brown with the Heart; then take out
the Lights, and add the Broth it was boiled in to
the Heart and Liver; and when there is no more
Gravy than what is ſufficient for Sauce, ſlice Half
of the Lights and add to it, and thicken the Gravy
with a little of thick melted Butter, and pour all
round the forced Liver. Lay Sippets round the Diſh,
and ſend it to the Table.

To make another Diſh of Veal's Pluck.

TAKE the Cat's-collop, and with a ſharp pointed Knife ſlit it open at one End down to the other; then force a Piece of the Liver as above, and ſtuff this Collop; ſew up the End, and ſet it in an Oven, or broil it before the Fire; and in the mean while cut half a Pound of Veal into thin Slices, and fry in a clean Haſh-pan, over a ſlow Stove with Butter; cut four Slices of the Liver and fry with the Veal; then put to it two Quarts of Water, an Onion ſtuck with four Cloves, Sweet-herbs, and a few Corns of Black-pepper; and when the Gravy is half conſumed, ſtrain it off; then take two Calf's-feet that has been boiled tender, take out their Bones, cut them in thin Slices, cut the other half of the Lights as above, and let them ſtew till there is no more Gravy than what is required for Sauce; then take the Cat's-collop and lay it in the Middle of the Haſh; fry ſome Liver, and lay round all with Raſhers of Bacon.

To make a Ragoo of Beef.

TAKE and cut four Pounds of the Rib-end of the Fore-crop next to the Chine, which is mixt like to a Neat's Tongue; ſeaſon it with Mace, Nutmeg, Pepper and Salt, and put it cloſe down into a Stew-pan or Pot, with a quarter of a Pound of Butter, a Pint of Water, a Head of Shalot, cover it cloſe, and let it ſtand three Hours in an Oven; then take a Pound of the Buttock of Bullock-Beef, and cut into thin Slices, and fry in a Haſh-pan brown with Butter: Then add to it three Pints of Water, ſome Sweet-marjoram and Thyme, and let it ſtew over a gentle Stove; then make ſome ſavoury Force-meat into round Balls, two Ox-palates boiled tender and cut into Dices, two Sweetbreads broiled brown and cut into ſquare Dices, four

Ar-

Artichoke-bottoms boiled and cut into four each, and a Spoonful of pickled Muſhrooms; when the Gravy is conſumed to a Pint, ſtrain it off and waſh the Pan; then put in all as above into the Stew-pan; and when the Beef has been the full Time in the Oven, take it out and put it in the Ragoo, and skim off all the Fat from the Gravy that the Beef was ſtewed in; ſtrain it and put it to the Ragoo, and let it ſtew till there is no more Gravy than is ſufficient for Sauce: Lay Sippets round the Diſh, and garniſh with green Pickles. Set the Beef in the Middle, and over it pour the Ragoo.

Beef *a la Mode.*

TAKE a thin ribby Piece of Beef next to the Bris-ket, bone and roll it cloſe up after ſeaſoning it with Mace, Cloves, Nutmeg, and Salt; then put it into a Stew-pot that will juſt hold it, and let it ſtand in an Oven all Night; then take Bones of the Beef and boil in three Quarts of Water, with a Bundle of Sweet-herbs and an Onion; then take a Pound of Veal and cut into thin Collops, and fry brown; and when one Half of the Broth the Beef-bones was boiled in is conſumed, ſtrain it into the Stew-pan to the fry'd Veal, and let it ſtew to a Pint; then boil a Hundred of large Aſparagus, ſtrain off the Gravy from the Veal, and cut the green Tops of the Graſs into Inch Lengths, and let them ſtew in the Gravy five Minutes: To keep the Beef hot you muſt keep it before a hot Fire, and pour the Gravy from it, and skim off all the Fat; then add the Beef-gravy to the Aſparagus, and boil it up: Toaſt ſome Bread and lay round the Diſh. Set the Beef in the Middle, pour over the ſtew'd Aſparagus, and ſend it up.

Dev'd

Dov'd Beef.

TAKE four or five Pounds of the Part of the Buttock of Beef, that has Fat at the Top, ſome calls it the Steek, ſtick ten Cloves all over, and ſet it into the Oven in a Stew-pot, with a Quarter of a Pound of Butter, and half a Pint of Water; then take two Pounds of the Buttock of Beef, and fry it in thin Slices with Butter in a Stew-pan brown, then add to it three Quarts of Water, and let it ſtew over the Stove; then take a Pound of Carrots, boil and cut them in Dices, and a Pound of Turnips half boil them, and cut one of them in the Form of carved Sippets and lay round the Diſh; cut the reſt of the Turnips in Dices, and ſtrain the Gravy when it is conſumed to a Pint, waſh the Pan clean and put the Turnips and Carrots with the Gravy into it; and when the Beef is tender take it out, skim off all the Fat, and ſtrain the Gravy to the Roots and let it boil: Then ſet the Beef on the Middle of the Diſh, your carved Sippets round, pour over your Roots and Gravy, and ſerve it up.

A ſtew'd Rump of Beef.

TAKE a Rump of Beef and bone it, put it into a broad Stewing-pot: Add to it a Quart of Water, Shalot, a Bundle of Sweet-herbs; then cover it, and paſte the Cover cloſe, ſo that no Steam can get out, and let it ſtand in a moderate Oven eight Hours; boil two Ox-palates ſix Hours of that Time, an Ounce of Truffles and Morels boiled tender, cut the Palates into ſmall Dices; then take the Beef out of the Stewing-pot, and skim off all the Fat from the Gravy, and ſet the Beef on a Soup-diſh, and ſtrain the Gravy into a Haſh-pan: Add the Palates, Truffles and Morels, and boil them one Minute; toaſt Bread and cut into Dices, and put it into the Diſh: Pour in the Soup and ſerve it up. By
this

this Receipt you may ſee what Strength is in Beef, and what it is able to do without Hot-ſpices: If the Beef be good, the Beef and Soup will have one Taſte, and by this Method any Part of the Beef may be done.

To ſtew an Ox Head.

TAKE a ſharp Knife and take off the Fleſh from the Bones, and waſh it through many warm Waters; ſeaſon it with Nutmeg, Pepper and Salt, and put it into a Stewing-pot: Add to it a Pint of ſtale Beer, two Heads of Shalot, a Bundle of Sweet-herbs; then break the Jaw-bones, lay over the Head, cover it cloſe, paſte it, and ſet it in the Oven all Night; and when you take it out, if it is very tender, put the Head into a Pot, and preſs it down with a Cover, ſtrain the Gravy into another Pot, and ſo cut ſome of the Head in Slices, to warm in a Haſh-pan with Part of the Gravy: Lay Sippets round the Diſh and ſend it up.

A made Diſh of Lamb.

TAKE a hind Quarter of Lamb and cut off the Leg, bone it, and cut ſome of the Lean out of the Leg; take the Fat of the Loin and ſome of the Lean, and ſhred very fine, and ſeaſon it with Nutmeg, Pepper and Salt; cut ſome green Thyme and Sweet-marjoram ſmall, and add to it grated Bread and two Eggs, ſtuff the Leg with this, and ſet it into an Oven in an Earthen-pot; then cut the Loin into Collops, and ſeaſon it with Nutmeg, Mace, Pepper and Salt; ſet on the Bones of the Leg and Loin to boil in a Quart of Water, ſtick an Onion with three Cloves, and boil it with the Sweet-herbs; then fry your Collops a light Brown, put them in a Haſh-pan, and when the Gravy is conſumed to a Jill, ſtrain it on the Collops, and add a Spoonful of pickled Muſhrooms: When the Leg of
Lamb

Lamb is enough take it out, pour off the Gravy, skim off the Fat, and put the Gravy into the Collops; tofs them up, pour them on the Difh, and fet the forced Leg in the Middle. Garnifh the Difh with green Pickles and ferve it up.

Stew'd Lambs Heads.

TAKE two Lambs Heads and fplit them, take out the Brains and Tongues whole, and wafh them very clean, boil them in a Stew-pan till tender; then take out the Heads, and cut a Pound of Veal into Collops, and fry them in a Stew-pan on a flow Fire with Butter till they are Brown, pour in the Broth the Heads were boil'd in; then take two half Heads, and with a Knife cut each a-crofs by way of Checker-work, and rub them over with the Yolk of an Egg; then ftrew over grated Bread and Parfley cut fmall, and fet them on a Tin-pan before the Fire, bafte them with Butter and crifp them; Strain off the Gravy, and wafh the Stew-pan, and put the Gravy and the two other Halfs into it; and while it is a ftewing, you may take out of the Brains all the red Strings that is on them; dip them in Egg, and ftrew over them fome grated Bread, and have fome boiling Fat and fry them in; then make up half a Pound of favoury Force-meat into Balls, and fry them; then add to the ftewed Head a Spoonful of Catchup, four Artichoke-bottoms cut in Quarters; and thicken the Sauce with Flour and Butter: Then fet your broiled Halfs oppofite to each other in the Difh, the ftewed Halfs the fame Way; and pour your Sauce in, and lay the Brains round the Difh with the Force-meat Balls, and ferve it up.

To ftew a Calf's Head.

CLEAVE the Head, and take out the Brains and Eyes; cut the Skull off and the grifly Part with the Mouth, and put it into a Stew-pot; feafon
with

with Mace, Nutmeg, and Pepper; add to it a Pint
of Water, a Quarter of a Pound of Butter, ſome
Shalot, and Sweet-herbs; cover it cloſe, paſte the
Cover that no Steam can get out; and three Hours
will do in a moderate Oven: And in the mean
Time fry a Pound of Buttock Beef cut into Collops
with Butter brown; then add to it a Quart or three
Pints of Water, and let it ſtew into a Pint; then
ſtrain it off, and clean your Pan; boil half a Hundred of Aſparagus, and cut the Tops in half Inches
long, and ſtew them in this Gravy; then dip the
Brains in Egg, and boil them in the above Manner:
Fry ſome Raſhers of the Flank Part of the Bacon;
take out the Head and lay it in the Diſh; skim off
all the Fat of the Gravy the Head was ſtew'd in;
add as much as you need to the Gravy and Aſparagus, and pour it over the Head; then lay the Brains
and Raſhers of Bacon round the Diſh, and ſerve it
up.

A rolled Breaſt *of* Veal.

TAKE a Breaſt of Veal and bone it, lay it out
its Length on the Table; ſeaſon it with Nutmeg, Pepper and Salt, green Thyme, Sweet-marjoram, and Parſley cut very ſmall, rub the Yolk of
Egg over the Inſide of it; then ſtrew on the Herbs,
and lay Force-meat over the Roll of Veal the long-
way, and bind it with Pack-thread; boil it in a Stew-
pan in as much Water as will cover it; and when
it boils down, turn it, ſo that it may boil equally;
when it is boiled thoroughly, pour off its Gravy, and
skim off all the Fat; clean waſh your Pan, and ſtrain
in the Gravy: Add to it a Jill of brown drawn Gravy, with two Veal Sweet-breads broiled and cut
each into ſix Parts, ſome Force-meat Balls, and a
few Muſhrooms: Cut the Breaſt in Three, let each
Part ſtand upright; lay carv'd Sippets and Lemon
round the Diſh; pour on the Gravy, and ſerve it up.

To dreſs Sheep Rumps.

TAKE eight Sheep Rumps and boil them tender; and take in the mean Time six Lamb-ſtones, and as many Suckles, and fry them Brown; then take ſome Puff-paſte, and with a Jager-iron, or what is commonly term'd Runners, cut this Puff-paſte into Strings as ſmall as Tape of three Yards a Penny; then rub each Rump with Yolk of Egg, and ſtrow over ſome Parſley cut ſmall; and take the Puff-paſte and lay on each Rump in the long-way, and croſs them with the Paſte, ſo as to make them a ſmall Diamond Figure, and ſet them in the Oven, which is to be a ſharp one; then take half a Pint of Gravy, fry to Force-meat Balls, and toſs up with the Lamb-ſtones and Suckles, adding a little thick drawn Butter: Toſs all together and pour on the Diſh, and lay the Rumps all round it.

To dreſs Hog's Feet *and* Ears.

TAKE a Gang of Hog's Feet and Ears and boil them tender; then cut off all the Fleſh from the Bones of the Feet, and cut it into Slices as for a Haſh; then ſeaſon it with Mace, Cloves, Nutmeg, Salt, and Pepper, and put it into a Stew-pan; add to it a Pint of brown Veal-gravy; and cut a Calf's Foot boil'd tender into thin Slices, and cut them in Pieces, and add to the Gravy and Feet: Then cut one Ear into thin Slices, and add to it the other cut in the ſame Form, dip them in Egg, and fry'd brown with Fat: Then cut pickled Cucumbers and lay round the Diſh; pour in the Stew, and lay the fry'd Ear all over it, and ſerve it up.

To Ragoo *a* Beef's Heart.

TAKE a Beef's Heart, and cut out the Inſide of the Meat, and lard it all over with Bacon; take a Pound of Beef-ſuet with a Quarter of a Pound

M of

of Meat you cut out of the Heart, ſhred it very fine, or beat it in a Mortar, and grate into it the Crumbs of a *French* Roll: Seaſon it with Nutmeg, Pepper, and Salt; cut ſmall ſome Cloves, Thyme, Parſley, and Sweet-marjoram; break into it two Eggs, and work it up with your Hand, and ſtuff the Heart with this Force-meat; ſet it with the Point of the Heart up in a Pot into an Oven, and cover the Pot; it will take two Hours and a Half baking: In which Time cut the Remainder of the Meat you took out of the Heart as thin as *Scotch* Collops; ſeaſon them with Nutmeg, Pepper, and Salt, and fry them in a Stew-pan with Butter; then add to them a Quart of ſtrong Broth, and let it ſtew, cut a Neat's Foot into thin Pieces, and add to it: When there is Gravy ſufficient for Sauce, and the Heart in the Oven the above Time, take it out, ſet it in the Middle of the Diſh, and pour over the Ragoo; throw Muſhrooms over, and lay Sippets round.

To a la mode a Calf's Head.

YOUR Calf's Head muſt have the Skin on, the Hair ſinged off with a hot Poker, and after ſcraped clean with a Knife; then with a very ſharp Pen-knife take the Head from the Bone, the Tongue taken out and boiled, the Head larded all over with Bacon, and fill'd with Force-meat made very ſtiff, and skewer'd in the full Height and Form it was in before, and put it into a long Pot that will hold it with Eaſe; cover and ſet it into an Oven three Hours; then take the Tongue and cut it into thin Slices, with two Sweet-breads fryed brown: And take three Jills of Beef-gravy and put into a Stew-pan, into which put the ſliced Tongue and Sweet-bread, each cut into eight Pieces; add to them ſome Muſhrooms, Truffles, and Morels, being firſt boiled tender in Water; and when the Gravy is conſumed by gentle ſtewing on a ſlow Fire, to as much as is ſufficient

ficient for Sauce, and the Head enough, take it out:
Garniſh your Diſh with carved Lemon and green
Pickles, pour on the Stew; ſet the Head in the
Middle, and ſerve it up.

Lamb *in Blankets.*

TAKE a Loin of Lamb, and take the Kidney
and Fat for Force-meat; cut the Fleſh the
long Way from the Chine, and make the Collop
half a Quarter ſquare, beat it, and make eight Collops of the above Size, and rub them over with Yolk
of Egg: Seaſon them with Nutmeg and Salt, and
lay a thin Lair of Force-meat, and roll it up: In
the ſame Manner do all the Eight. Then break
ſix Ounces of Butter into three Pints of Flour very
ſmall, work the Butter in the Flour, then beat up
two Eggs with a Jill of fair Water; make a Paſte
of this Flour and Butter, and roll out eight Sheets,
into each one roll up a Roll of Lamb, and tye a
Cloth over every one at each End, and have a Stew-
pan of boiling Water ready, into which put your
Lamb, let them boil a full Hour: For Sauce, have
Gravy and Butter: Take them out of the Clothes,
lay them round the Diſh, and pour over the Sauce.
Garniſh with Puff-paſte baked, and Sippets.

To Ragoo a Shoulder *of* Lamb.

TAKE a well grown Fore-quarter of Lamb, and
cut off the Shoulder cloſe to the Breaſt; with
a Knife cut open the Shoulder at the broad End,
take out the Shull and Shank-bones, but take Care
not to break through on either Side; then ſtuff the
Places where the Bones were taken out with Force-
meat; lay the Shoulder on an Earthen-diſh, and ſet
it in an Oven an Hour: Then take ſix Lamb-ſtones
and eight Suckles, ſplit the Stones, ſeaſon them with
Nutmeg, Pepper and Salt; fry them brown, and

M 2 put

put them in a Stew-pan; adding a Pint of Gravy, ſome Muſhrooms, a Quarter of a Hundred of Aſparagus boiled tender; cut off the green Tops, and add to the Suckles and Stones: When the Shoulder is enough take it out, pour off all the Fat; put the Gravy into the Stew-pan, and let it boil with the Ragoo one Minute; then lay the Shoulder in the Middle of the Diſh, and pour over it the Ragoo: Lay green Pickles round the Diſh, and ſerve it up.

Minced Beef Collops.

CUT a Pound and a Half out of the Fillet; the Part of the Sirloin that lies next the Chine under the Suet, mince this as ſmall as minced Veal; take the Marrow of two Beef-bones, cut ſmall, and mix it with the minced Collops: Then fry them in a Pan over a ſlow Fire; ſeaſon them with a little Pepper and Salt, keep them ſtirring all the Time: Lay toaſted Bread round the Diſh, and have no Sauce but the Marrow and themſelves.

Broiled Beef Collops.

CUT Stakes off the Rump of Bullock-beef half an Inch thick; have a very clear Fire and a clean hot Grate-iron, lay two Stakes on at a Time, and keep them frequently turning; when the Stakes are rather hard, they will be enough: Then lay them on a hot Diſh, with ſcraped Horſe-raddiſh. If you obſerve the Directions, the Beef-ſtakes will diſcharge more Gravy than needful for Sauce.

To make Veal Cutlets.

TAKE a Neck of fine Veal, cut a Rib to every Cutlet, and flat them with the Side of a Bill-knife; then ſeaſon them with Mace, Nutmeg, Pepper and Salt; rub each Cutlet with the Yolk of Eggs, grate ſome Bread, and roll each Cutlet in it;

have

have ſome clean Beef-fat boiling hot in a Haſh-pan on a Stove, and fry them very quickly on it: For Sauce, have ſome Butter, Gravy, and Muſhrooms; pour it into a hot Diſh, lay the Cutlets criſp and hot on the Sauce, with Lemon round the Diſh, and ſerve it up.

To make a Pellow.

IF you boil a Knockle of Veal, take Care your Pot be very clean; put no more Water than will cover it, with a little White-pepper, and three Blades of Mace; when the Veal is enough boiled, ſtrain off the Broth into an Earthen-pot, and let it ſtand all Night; then skim off all the Top, and take two Quarts of this Broth into a large Sauce-pan, ſet it on the Fire, and when it boils, put in a large Fowl; be ſure to skim it very well when it boils: Then add to it three Quarters of a Pound of Rice, let it boil till the Fowl is tender, and the Rice ſeems thick; then take up the Fowl, and add a Jill of thick Cream to the Rice; when it boils, cover the Fowl with Rice, and pour the Remainder into the Diſh: Lay boiled Spinnage round the Diſh-edge, by Way of Garniſhing.

Turkey *a la Royal.*

TAKE a Turkey after it is well pick'd and ſing'd, cut it down the Back, and bone it, only leave the Pinions on, and lard it all over with Bacon; make ſavoury Force-meat, and fill the Places where you took out the Bones; put into the Body and Crop a Pound and a Half of Force-meat, ſew the Back up again with ſtrong Thread, leaving a Piece of the Thread to pull out the Reſt by, when it is ready to ſend to Table: Skewer it in the ſame Form as for roaſting: Then ſet it on a deep Earthen-diſh, and ſet it two Hours in an Oven; cover it over

with

with a Sheet of Cap-paper well butter'd: For
Sauce, take a Jill of brown Veal-gravy, and take
off the Beards of 30 Oyſters, after you have plumpt
them; then add a Spoonful of pickled Muſhrooms.
When you take out your Turkey, skim all the Fat
off the Gravy, that is in the Diſh it was baked
in; add this Gravy to your Sauce: Lay carved
Lemon and Sippets round the Diſh, pour on your
Sauce, and ſet on your Turkey. Remember to pull
out the Thread you ſewed up the Back.

To a la mode a Goose.

AFTER your Gooſe is well picked and ſinged,
cut it down the Back, and bone it in the above
Manner; make two Pounds of Force-meat, and
ſtuff it with; ſew up the Back as aforeſaid, and
with a ſharp Knife make checkered Work on the
Breaſt of it; lay it on a flat-bottom'd Diſh, and
rub it all over with the Yolk of Egg; then ſtrew
on grated Bread and ſome Butter; ſet it three Hours
in the Oven: For Sauce, have a Jill of Gravy, and
a Jill of ſcalded Gooſe-berries, which pour into the
Diſh; ſet the Gooſe on the Middle, and ſerve it up.

To a la mode Fowls.

TAKE three young Pouts and bone them, put a
Quarter of a Pound of Force-meat into every
Fowl, but they are not to be cut down the Backs,
the Bones are to be taken out at the Neck-end of
them; when they are equally ſtuffed, put every
Fowl into a Bladder, and boil them an Hour: Lay
Puff-paſte, Sippets, and carved Lemon round the
Diſh: For Sauce, have ſome white Veal-gravy and
Muſhrooms, ſix Yolks of Eggs hard boil'd whole;
thicken it with Flour and Butter. Take out the
Fowls, ſet them on the Diſh, pour on the Sauce,
and ſerve them up.

Chickens

Chickens *a la Royal.*

TAKE four large Chickens, pick, singe, and clean them well, cut them down the Back, and bone them; take half a Pound of Marrow, half a Pound of Beef-suet, and half a Pound of the Flesh of a Fowl, with grated Bread, Eggs, and Seasoning into a Force-meat, stuff them, lard them with Bacon, sew up their Backs, and skewer them as if for roasting, leave on their Pinions; lay them on a flat-bottomed Earthen-dish, and set them in an Oven: Boil half a Hundred of Asparagus-tops tender, and cut into half Inch Lengths; take a Jill of brown Veal-gravy, and boil the Grass up in it, thicken it with Butter and Flour; then take out your Chickens, and set on the Dish. Garnish with carved Lemon, and pickled Kidney-beans.

A Ragoo of young Ducks.

KILL three young Ducks, pick, singe, and bone them well; stuff them with savoury Force-meat, let the Feet be kept on, and take off their Stockings; put in each three small Skewers at an equal Distance from each other, to keep them as in the Form for roasting: Then take a Stew-pan, and set it on a slow Stove, with four Ounces of Butter, and melt it; then flour your Ducks, and fry them brown; adding a Quart of Veal-broth, and let them stew with their Livers, Gizzards, and Pinions, an Onion, and Sweet-herbs; and when half of the Gravy is consumed, take out the Ducks, strain it, and skim off the Fat; boil a Pint of green Peas in Water, and drain them through a Hair-sieve; then put them to the Gravy that the Ducks were stewed in, and keep it on the Stove till it boils, then put in the Ducks; squeeze in the Juice of a Lemon, pour in half a Jill of thick melted Butter, toss all well together, and serve them up.

A

A *jugg'd* Hare.

SKIN your Hare and cut it into Joints, season it with Mace, Nutmeg, Pepper and Salt; clap it close in an Earthen-mug, and lay over it half a Pound of sweet Butter; then cover it close, paste it down, and set it three Hours in an Oven: Take its Liver, with a Quarter of a Pound of Beef-suet shred very fine, or beat in a Marble Mortar; add Shalot, green Thyme, Parsley, Sweet-marjoram, Nutmeg, Pepper and Salt, the Crumb of a Half-penny Roll steep'd in Milk; then squeeze out the Milk, and take the Bread and an Egg, mix all together; flour a Piece of Linen Cloth, and put this Pudding into it, tye it up, and boil it: Then take the Head of the Hare, and rub it over with the Yolk of Egg, baste it with melted Butter, then grate Bread over it, and set it into the Oven: When the Hare is enough, that is, when it has been in the Oven the above Time, take it out, and pour from it all the Gravy; add to it half a Jill of Beef-gravy, and thicken it with Butter and Flour: Then lay Sippets round the Dish, into which lay the Hare; pour over the Gravy, cut the Pudding in Slices, and lay all over; set the Head in the Middle, and send it up to Table.

Cocks-combed Tripes.

TO cocks-combed Tripes, you must have an Iron made in the Shape of a Cocks-comb, and take the lean Part of the finest Tripe you can get; cut out a Pound of Cocks-combs, and have three Jills of Beef-gravy, into which put your Cocks-combs, and let them stew; then cut the thick Part of a Bullock's-foot into thin Dices, and add to them; cut a Piece of the Double-round, and dip it in Batter; cut some of the thin Tripe, in the Shape of half a Crown, and ten of these fry Brown: Then

toss

toſs up the Cocks-combs, with a little Vinegar and Muſtard, and pour them on to the Diſh : Lay the Double-tripe in the Middle, and the other round it. Garniſh with pickled Onions, and Barberry-berries.

To fry Tripes.

WASH and dry your Tripes well, make a Batter of an Egg, a Spoonful of Flour, and three Spoonfuls of Milk beat very ſmooth; then dip in your Tripe, and have ready ſome fine Beef-fat boiling, and fry the Tripe a fine criſp light brown : For Sauce, melted Butter and Muſtard.

To fry Neat's Feet.

TAKE all the Bones out of the Bullock's Feet, and cut in Pieces the Length of your Finger, and the Breadth of Two; make the aforeſaid Batter, and dip each Piece, frying it in Fat as for Tripes : For Sauce, Muſtard, melted Butter and Vinegar.

Caſed Veal Cutlets.

CUT out of a Leg of Veal twelve thin Collops, let them be a direct Square; ſeaſon them with Mace, Nutmeg, and Salt; rub them over with Yolk of Egg, grate ſome Bread and throw on each Side of them, and make for each a Sheet of Puff-paſte no thicker than Wafer, paper cloſe round the Sides of the Cutlets, and ſet them in a Tin-pan into a hot Oven: If the Oven is equally hot Top and Bottom, they will be done in ten Minutes, and will be ſavoury and criſp, and is ſent up without Sauce. This Way is very much liked by Ladies and Gentlemen of weak Conſtitutions and tender Stomachs.

To

To dreſs a Calf's Head.

TAKE out the Eyes and ſplit the Head, take out the Brains, waſh the Head in warm Water, and afterwards in cold Water, till it is very clean, and then boil it; when it is enough, take it up and cut it a-croſs with a ſharp Knife till you make Dice-work of each Side; then rub it over with Yolk of Egg, throw on ſome grated Bread, and ſet it in a Tin-pan before the Fire; but if you have an Oven rather uſe it, only you muſt baſte with melted Butter before you put it in, and let it ſtand till it is brown: For Sauce, boil the Brains and mix with melted Butter, and a Spoonful of Vinegar. Set on the two Halfs upright in the Diſh, lay broiled Raſhers of Bacon all over the Skull, and round the Diſh; then ſerve it up.

To roaſt a Pig like Lamb.

TAKE a fat Pig and kill it, take off the Hair and skin it, cut it into Quarters and draw it with Parſley: Take the Skin and Head of it; take the Bones out of two Rabbets, rub the Inſide of the Pig with Yolk of Eggs, and join the Rabbets cloſe to the Skin of the Pig; take the Bottom of a long *French* Roll, take out the Crumb, put a clean Rag within the Roll to keep it up, fix the Roll to the Pig's Head, and lay it in the Inſide of the Pig; then turn them over into a Tin-pan, and ſet it into an Oven, with Flour drudged over it; when it is near done, take it out, and wipe off the Flour with a clean Wing of a Gooſe, rub it all over with clean Feathers dipt in melted Butter, throw Salt over it, and ſet it into an Oven till it is enough; then have in readineſs a Jill of Gravy, with a little boiled Sage in it; draw the Pig, and with a clean Wing duſt all the Salt off it; take the Cloth out of the Roll,
ſend

ſend it up Whole to the Table; let the Roll ſtay within it, and pour the Gravy into the Diſh. So you have four Quarters of a Pig and a whole one, out of one Pig, by the Art of Cookery and a little Help.

A Made-diſh of Sheep Heads *and* Tongues.

TAKE two good Weather Heads and eight Tongues, waſh your Heads well after you have ſplit them and taken their Eyes out; put them into a Pot with juſt as much Water as will cover them, and take Care of all the Brains; waſh all the Tongues, and boil them with the Heads: Take a Pound of Veal and cut into thin Collops, fry them brown on a ſlow Stove, in a Haſh-pan; then take up the Heads and Tongues, ſtrain three Pints of the Broth into the Haſh-pan, and let it boil; then take the eight Tongues, lard and blanch them with Bacon, pick the Fleſh clean from the Bone of the Heads, and take great Care to keep it whole, *viz.* not to break through, and disfigure the half Face of the Sheep: Then ſeaſon the Heads with Mace, Nutmeg, Pepper, and Herbs cut very ſmall; roll out a Sheet of Puff-paſte as thin as Wafer-paſte, cover each Side of the Sheep's Face with it, and ſet it in the Oven: Take out the larded Tongues and ſtrain off the Gravy, waſh your Pan clean, put in your Gravy and Tongues; add to them ſome Muſhrooms, Truffles and Morels ſtew'd tender, 20 Force-meat Balls, dip the Brains in Egg and fry them in hot Fat: Toſs all up, lay the Tongues round the Diſh, pour on the Gravy, Balls, and Muſhrooms; ſet the Heads in the Middle, the Brains all over, ſo ſerve it up. This is a Head-diſh for a firſt Courſe.

N

A Made-dish of Sweet-breads.

TAKE four Sweet-breads, and season with Nutmeg and Salt; one of the Largest rub over
with Yolk of Egg, grate Bread, roll it on, and broil
it before the Fire; season the other Three, and fry
them brown with Butter; take a Pint of brown
Veal-gravy, cut the three Sweet-breads into Dices,
and put them into the Gravy to stew; boil eight
Eggs hard, and take out the Yolks whole: When
the Gravy is consumed to what is sufficient for
Sauce, add to it a little melted Butter, and toss
it up. Lay Sippets and carved Lemon round the
Dish, pour on the stew'd Sweet-breads, lay the
broiled one in the Middle, with Yolk of Eggs all
over, and serve it up.

A boiled Turkey.

BOIL your Turkey in Oat-meat and Water; take
Sellery and cut in Pieces no larger than the
Breadth of your Finger; take a Pint of White-gravy
of Veal, and put to it a Pint of cut Sellery, let it
stew till the Sellery is tender, then grate in a little
Nutmeg and Salt, add to it some plain melted Butter:
And when the Turkey is enough, take it up and set
it on a Dish; pour over your Sauce, and garnish
your Dish with carved Lemon.

A boiled Turkey with Rice.

SKEWER your Turkey for boiling, and take a
Quarter of a Pound of Beef-suet, and the Crumbs
of a Halfpenny Roll grated, a little Nutmeg and
Egg work'd up together with your Hand, put it
into the Turkey's Crop, sew it up, and put it into
a Pot and boil it; then take half a Pound of Rice
and boil tender in Water, and when it begins to
thicken

thicken, take a Quarter of a Pound of Butter and toſs
it up with, adding a little Nutmeg and Salt to it:
Set the Turkey on a Diſh, and ſmother it with Rice;
pour the Remainder on the Diſh and ſerve it up.

A boiled Turkey *and* Oyſter *Sauce.*

PUT your Turkey up for boiling, and grate the
Crumb of a Penny *French* Roll; take a Slice of
ſweet Butter and work up in the Crumbs, grate Nutmeg and Salt: Add an Egg, and ſtuff a little Thyme,
Parſley, and Sweet-marjoram cut very ſmall; work
all well together, and ſtuff the Crop of the Turkey,
ſew it up, and boil it; then take half a Hundred of
good freſh Oyſters, and put them a Minute or two
on the Fire to plump, and take one by one out
of their Liquor; then melt a Quarter of a Pound of
Butter, into which put your Oyſters with a little
of their Liquor: Add a little White-wine, Nutmeg,
a very little Bread boiled in Water, toſs up all very
well; take up your Turkey, and lay it in your Diſh,
and pour on your Oyſter-ſauce: Lay Sippets round
Diſh and carved Lemon, ſo ſend it up.

A boiled Fowl *ſmother'd with* Onions.

PUT up your Fowl for boiling, and let it be well
ſinged; after rub it very well, waſh and dry it;
then duſt a little Flour over it, boil it in ſoft Water, it will be white if you do not over-boil it; and
boil ſix large Onions very ſoft, beat them to Pulp,
and mix them with melted Butter: Lay the Fowl
on a Diſh, and pour over the Onion-ſauce. The
ſame Sauce is made for boiled Rabbets.

To make a Veniſon Paſty.

BONE your Veniſon and ſeaſon it with Black-
pepper and Salt, put it in a Pot and cover it
cloſe; ſet it two Hours in an Oven, put into the
Pot

Pot over it, half a Pound of ſweet Butter, and accord-to the Size of your Paſty-pan make a Quantity of Paſte; break two Pounds of Butter into four Pounds of Flour, mix it with cold Water to a Paſte; cut a Pound of Butter into Slices and lay over the Paſte, drudge Flour over the Butter, and roll it out three Times, drudging Flour each Time, cover the Inside and Edges of the Pan; take the Veniſon out of the Oven, and put into it, and if it wants Fat, take the fat Laps of a good Shoulder of Weather mutton and lay over it; then lay over all a Sheet of paste, and cut out Leaves and Flowers on the Top of the Paſty: Two Hours will bake it; have a Pint of rich Gravy in Readineſs to pour into the [ ] ſoon as it comes out of the Oven, and ſend it up.

A Mutton Paſty.

TAKE a hind Quarter of little *Scotch* Mutton, bone and skin it, and bake it in an Oven in the aforeſaid Manner; put it in a Paſty-pan, as is di-rected; and give it the ſame Time to bake in: It will not be much inferior to a Veniſon Paſty.

A Florentine.

TAKE two Bullock's Feet and take out all the Bones, ſhred the Meat very ſmall, as if for minced Pyes; blanch a Pound of *Jourdan* Almonds, and mince ſmall with the Feet, ſtone half a Pound of Raſins and cut ſmall, a Pound and a half of Cur-rants well picked and waſhed, a Pound of Apples cut ſmall, and half a Pound of Sugar; ſeaſon with Mace, Cinnamon, and Nutmeg; make Paſty-paſte and lay round the Diſh-edge, and put in your minced Meat, mixing it well; then cover it with a Sheet of Paſte, and cut out your Florentine: Bake it two Hours, and ſerve it up.

A

A *Sweet* Veal Pye.

CUT a Loin of Veal into Chops, and season it
with Nutmeg, *Jamaica* Pepper, and Salt; take
half a Pound of Currants, half a Pound of Rasins
stoned, and a Quarter of a Pound of Almonds; take
Part of the Kidney-fat, shred it small or beat in a
Mortar, and some grated Bread; season it with Nutmeg and Salt, add Currants and, an Egg, and mix
all up into round Balls; then lay a Lair of Veal, and
upon that strew Fruit and Almonds, then another Lair
of Veal, and upon that strew Fruit and Almonds,
lay over that the Force-meat Balls, cover up your
Pye, and bake it an Hour and a half in an Oven;
make a Caudle of a Jill of Cream, with a little Butter, half a Jill of White-wine, and a little Sugar.
You may make a sweet Lamb Pye after the same
Manner.

A Mutton Pye.

TAKE a Neck of Mutton and cut into Chops,
scrape some small Potatoes, and season your
Chops with Pepper and Salt, and lay a Rim of
Paste round a Soup-dish; then lay a Lair of Mutton, and on that Potatoes, cover the Potatoes with
the rest of the Mutton, and fill up the Dish with
the rest of the Potatoes, put a Pint of Water into
the Dish and cover it up: It will take two Hours
Baking.

A Hare Pye.

BONE a Hare, and make a Pudding for her of
the Liver, a Quarter of a Pound of Beef-suet,
some grated Bread, and an Egg; season with Nutmeg, Pepper, and Salt; cut Thyme, Parsley, Sweet-
marjoram very small, and a little Shalot; mix these
with the Pudding, and put it into the Hare; raise
a standing Crust for it, and model your Paste into
the

the Shape of a Hare, ſet the Hare on her Belly as
ſhe is in her natural Seat: When you take off the
Skin, skin the Ears, and ſet her with her Head
down, and her Ears between her Shoulders; if you
are an expert Paſtry-cook make the Figure of the
Hare on the Lid of the Pye: Let her have two
Hours and a half baking; pour into your Pye as
ſoon as taken out of the Oven, a Pint of Veal
Gravy that Spices have been boiled in, and ſend
it up.

An Alio *of ſmall* Birds.

TAKE two Dozen of ſmall Birds and pick clean,
make a Force-meat of the Marrow of a Beef-
bone, and the Breaſt of a Fowl, beat in a Marble
Mortar, or ſhred very fine on a Board; ſeaſon with
Mace, Nutmeg, and Salt; take the Crumbs of a
Half-penny Roll and ſoak in Cream, and an Egg,
mix all well together; boil two Beef-palates tender,
and cut into ſmall Squares; then ſeaſon the Birds and
Palates with Nutmeg and Salt; lay the Birds into
a raiſed Cruſt not above three Inches high, lay the
Palates between the Birds, and ſpread the Force-
meat all over: An Hour will bake it; have in Readi-
neſs half a Pint of Veal-gravy, and pour into it as
ſoon as it is taken out of the Oven.

A Chicken Pye.

TAKE five young Chickens and skin them very
clean, grate a Nutmeg and mix with Salt; take
a Quarter of a Pound of Butter and mix with the
Nutmeg and Salt, and divide it into five Parts; take
out the Breaſt-bones of the Chickens, put them up
as for boiling, cut off their Legs, put into each
Chicken a Part of the Butter, lay them into a Diſh
or a Baker that juſt holds them, turn their Breaſts
down, lay Puff-paſte round the Sides of the Diſh
or

or Baker, cover it with Puff-paſte, and bake it in an Oven an Hour; then boil half a Hundred of Aſparagus in Water, cut them into half Inch Lengths, have ſome Veal-gravy ready, and ſtew them in the Gravy a Quarter of an Hour; then take the Lid off the Chickens, and turn the Breaſts up, and pour on the ſtewed Aſparagus and Gravy.

A Beef-ſtake Pye.

TAKE two Pounds of Beef out of the Fore-chine, that lies next to the Ribby-end, cut it very thin; ſeaſon with Mace, Nutmeg, Pepper, and Salt; boil three Ox-palates tender, and cut ſmall; make Paſty-paſte, roll it out, and lay a Paſte round the Rim of the Diſh; lay in your Beef-ſtakes, and the Palates between the Stakes, add three Slices of Butter, and cover them with the Paſte: Bake the Pye two Hours, and when you take it out of the Oven, pour into it half a Pint of ſtrong Broth, and ſend it up.

A Mutton-ſtake Pye.

CUT out the Part of a Leg of Mutton where the Pope's Eye is, and cut it round, ſo that the Pope's Eye may appear in the Middle, the Mutton round it as a Border, and cut the Slices thin; take a Pound of very ſmall Kidney-potatoes and ſcrape them; ſeaſon the Mutton with Pepper and Salt; lay a Lair of Mutton, and a Lair of Potatoes till your Diſh is full, cover it with thin Slices of Butter, and make the aforeſaid Paſte in the above Manner: Bake it, and when it is enough pour in a Pint of Mutton-gravy, and ſend it up.

A Duck Pye.

BONE a Couple of Ducks, and after you have picked and ſinged them well, waſh them clean,
O   and

and dry them with clean Towels; take a Pound of white Force-meat made of the Breaſts of Fowls, Beef-ſuet, and grated Bread; ſeaſon it with Nutmeg, Pepper and Salt, Thyme, Sweet-marjoram, and Parſley cut ſmall, and work it up with an Egg; rub the Inſide of the Ducks with the Yolk of an Egg, and lay a thin Lair of Force-meat upon it; put the Ducks in their natural Form, and raiſe an ovel Cruſt, into which lay the Ducks, and lid the Pye: Bake it two Hour, in which Time make ſome brown Gravy:- Add to it a Veal's-ſuckle cut into eight Parts, two Artichoke-bottoms cut into Quarters; when the Pye is baked cut up the Lid, boil up the Gravy and pour over the Ducks, and ſend it up.

A Ham Pye.

TAKE a two Years old well cured Ham, and lay it in cold Water all Night, or twelve Hours; then take it out, take off all the Skin, cut off the ruſly Part of the under Side of it with a ſharp Knife; then put it into a long Earthen-pot that will juſt hold it, and lay it with the fat Side uppermoſt; then put to it two Bottles of rough Cider, cover it cloſe, and ſet it in an Oven an Hour and a half; raiſe a Cruſt in the Shape of the Ham, as thick as the Walls of a Gooſe Pye, into which put the whole Ham; lid the Pye, and ſet it in an Oven two Hours and a half; in which Time make a Ragoo of ſtrong Gravy, two Veal-ſuckles broil'd and cut in Dices, ſix Artichoke-bottoms cut in Quarters, Force-meat Balls, Truffles and Morels boiled tender, and Muſhrooms, and toſs up the Ragoo; when you take out the Pye cut up the Lid, and pour it over the Ham; ornament it with various Shapes of Paſte cut out, as wild Beaſts, and Flowers: Send it up without the Lid.

A

A Chriſtmas Gooſe Pye.

TAKE a Stone of Flour, and boil up four Pounds
of Butter in three Quarts of Water, and mix
the Flour with the Butter firſt; then take as much
of the Water as will mix the other Part of the
Flour, work it well together, and when it is cool
raiſe an ovel Cruſt; then take a fat Gooſe and a
Turkey, pick off all the Feathers, clean and cut up
their Backs, and take out all their Bones; take a
Bullock's Tongue, blanch and ſplit it; ſeaſon the
Turkey and Gooſe with Nutmeg, *Jamaica* and
Black-pepper: Lay the Turkey on the Bottom of
the Pye, and upon it the ſplit Tongue, cover it
with the Gooſe; lay over the Gooſe all the Seam,
that is the Fat you took out of her; and make a
thick Lid, cover the Pye, and paper it well: It will
take ſix Hours baking; when you take it out of the
Oven, pour into it a Pound of melted Butter, and
ſet upon a cold Stone till it is cool.

An Ox Cheek Pye.

BONE an Ox Cheek and waſh it in many Waters, dry it with a clean Cloth, and ſeaſon it
with Black and *Jamaica* Pepper, and Salt; put it
into a Pot, and put a Jill of Claret to it, cover it
cloſe, paſting it ſo that no Steam can get out, and
ſet it four Hours in an Oven; then make Paſty-paſte,
and lay a Sheet round the Edge of a Soup-diſh;
take the Ox Cheek whole out of the Pot it was
baked in, and put it into the Soup-diſh: Add to it
a Quarter of a Pound of Butter, lay on it a thick
Sheet of Paſte, and bake it two Hours in an Oven;
make a Pint of ſtrong Beef-gravy, with a Jill of
the Liquor the Head was firſt ſtewed in, and when
it is taken out of the Oven, pour this into the Pye,
ſhake it well and ſend it up: This eats very much

like

like Veniſon, and has been taken for Veniſon by tolerable Judges.

A *Sweet* Mutton Pye.

TAKE a Loin of Mutton and take off the Skin, cut the thin Flank Part off it, and cut the Chine Part into Chops; ſeaſon it with *Jamaica* and Black-pepper, and Nutmeg; take half a Pound of Currants, and half a Pound of Raſins, ſtone the Raſins, pick the Currants, waſh them and dry them with a Cloth; take a Quarter of a Pound of Sugar; then lay a Lair of Mutton, upon which lay Fruit and Sugar, cover the Fruit with Mutton, and ſtrow over the Remainder of the Fruit and Sugar; then put in a Pint of Water, ſo cover the Diſh with Paſte, and bake it two Hours.

A *Savoury* Turbot Pye.

TAKE two Pounds of Turbot and cut a Pound and a half into thick Slices; ſeaſon it with Nutmeg, Pepper and Salt; make a raiſed Cruſt very thin, lay in your Turbot, lay on it a Quarter of a Pound of Butter, lid the Pye, and bake it an Hour and a half; in which Time cut the other Half into thin Slices, and fry brown with Butter in a little Haſh-pan, and add to it a Quart of Water; then take half a Hundred of Oyſters, heat them in a Sauce-pan, take off their Beards, and when the Fiſh-gravy is two Parts conſumed, ſtrain it into a Sauce-pan: Add to it the Oyſters with a little of the Liquor, a Spoonful of Catchup, and a Spoonful of Walnut Liquor; work a Piece of Butter and Flour, and thicken it up; ſet it on the Fire till it boils, and toſs it up; when the Pye has been the above Time in the Oven, take it out, cut up the Lid, pour in the Oyſters and Gravy, lay on the Lid, and ſerve it up.

A

A *Sweet* Turbot Pye.

TAKE a Pound and a half of Turbot and cut into thin Slices; season with Nutmeg, Mace and
Salt; take half a Pound of Currants, wash and pick
them, and half a Pound of Rasins, stone them; make
a Puff-paste Crust, lay Paste round the Sides of the
Dish, lay a Lair of Turbot, and cover it with Fruit;
then cover the Fruit with Turbot, and on it strew
the Remainder of the Fruit, and lay over all a Quarter of a Pound of Butter, then fix on the Lid; one
Hour will bake it: And when it comes out of the
Oven, make a Caudle of melted Butter and Sugar,
and half a Jill of White-wine, and pour into the Pye
after you have cut up the Lid, and send it up.

A Salmon Pye.

TAKE a Joul of Salmon and cut into thin Slices,
take half a Jill of Verjuice, and rub over each
Piece of Salmon; season it with *Jamaica* and Black-
pepper, Nutmeg and Salt; roll each Piece, and set
round the Bottom of a raised Crust, lay on the
Lid, and bake it two Hours; boil the Bones of the
Salmon, and fry four Slices in Butter; and when is
is fried brown, pour in the Fish Broth, and boil it
with the fried Salmon till it is something strong;
then take a Jill of Gooseberries, pick and scald them
in Water, add them to the Gravy, and some melted
Butter; and when you have taken the Pye out of
the Oven, cut the Lid up and take it off, and pour
over all the Salmon the Gravy and Gooseberries;
cut the Lid in eight Parts, and set round the Inside
of the Pye, and send to Table.

A Eel Pye.

TAKE eight large Eels, skin and wash them
clean, open and split them down the Middle,

and

and take out their Back-bones; feafon them with Nutmeg, Pepper and Salt, and put them into an Earthen-pot, put three Spoonfuls of Butter over them, cover them clofe, and fet them in an Oven four Hours, in which Time the Bones of the Eels will diffolve; then lay a Sheet of Puff-pafte all over the Difh that will juft hold them, and put them clofe; obferve to roll them as if for collaring, before you put them in the Pot; then lay a very thin Cover of Pafte over them, and let them bake an Hour: In which Time fet their Heads and Back-bones on the Fire with a Pint of Water, and let it boil to a Jill; then add to it a Spoonful of Catchup, thicken it with Butter and Flour; take out the Pye, pour in the Gravy, and fet it upon the Table.

An Oyfter Pye.

TAKE a Rock Codling and cut out the Back-bone, lay it in an Earthen-pan, pour upon it a Pint of White-wine or Goosberry-vinegar, and let it lie an Hour; then make a Pafty-pafte Cruft, and lay it very thin round the Difh; cut the Skin off the Fifh, take out all its Bones, and cut it in Pieces no larger than your Finger; then feafon it with Mace, Nutmeg, Pepper and Salt, and lay it into your Difh, with a Quarter of a Pound of Butter over it and a thin Pafte, and bake it an Hour in an Oven: Then take a Haddock and cut down the Middle, after it is cleaned, fry it brown in Butter, with the Tail of the Codling, in a Hafh-pan; adding to it a Quart of Water and the Bones of the Codling; when it is confumed to little above a Jill, ftrain through a Hair-fieve: Take 100 of Oyfters, fcald them, take off all their Beards, and put them into a Sauce-pan with the Fifh-gravy, and let them juft boil: Then take the Pye out of the Oven, cut up the Lid and take it off, pour all the Oyfters over

the

the Pye; cut the Lid into ſix Pieces, ſet them round, and ſend it up.

An Apple Cuſtard Pye.

LAY a Puff-paſte Cruſt all over a Baker, peel and core as many Apples as will fill it, put in Sugar and cover it, and bake it an Hour and a Half in an Oven; then take a Pint of Cream and boil it on the Fire with a Stick of Cinnamon, and ſet it to cool; then beat the Yolks of ſix Eggs very well, mix with the Cream, and ſweeten to your Taſte: Take out the Pye, cut up the Lid and take it off, and with the Back of your Spoon put down the Apples, and make it ſmooth; then pour over the Cream and Yolks of Eggs, and ſet it in five Minutes; then take it out, cut the Lid into Sippets and ſet round the Cuſtard; ſend it up to the Table cold. In all Apple Pyes be ſure to put in Lemon-skin cut ſmall.

A Cherry Pye.

LAY Puff-paſte all over a Baker, fill it with ſtoned Cherries, and ſweeten it to your Taſte; then roll out the Remainder of your Paſte, and cut it in Lengths to reach over the Pye; make each Piece into half Inch-breadths, and lay them croſs and croſs, to make them into Diamonds: Then ſet it into the Oven, take great Care to bake it beautiful, and ſend it up cold.

N. B. All Sweet-meat Pyes are to have open Lids, ſuch as Damſens, Plumbs, &c. and to be ſent up cold; or, red, white or black Currants in the ſame Manner; likewiſe Raſps and Strawberries.

A French Bean Pye.

TAKE a Quart of *French* blanched Beans, lay Puff-paſte over a Diſh-edge, boil eight Eggs
hard

hard, take out their Yolks whole, and lay all over
the Top of the Beans, likewiſe a Quarter of a Pound
of Sugar and the ſame of Butter, cover it up and
bake it an Hour: Then take a Jill of melted Butter
and half a Jill of Rheniſh, ſweeten it to your Taſte,
and pour it on.

To dreſs a Cod's Head.

CUT three Inches of the Cod's Shoulder towards
the Head, then rub the Head all over with very
ſtrong Vinegar, and cover it with Salt an Hour before you put it in to boil, and have hard Water to
boil it, let the Fire be very good, for it muſt boil
very faſt an Hour; skin eight Whitings and dip in
Batter, and fry in clarified Butter; drain the Head
over the Water it was boiled in, and while it is
draining, take off all the black Skin; when the Fiſh
is boiling, break a Lobſter and take out all the
Meat, cut it ſmall, and boil it up in melted Butter,
grate on ſome Nutmeg, add Catchup, Red-wine, of
each a Spoonful; cut ſome of the Liver and dip into Batter, fry it; then take the long ſmall Bones
out of the Jaw Fins of the Head, and ſtick on each
End Muſhrooms, Oyſters, Barberryberry; ſet the
Head on a Diſh, and let it be hot, lay your forced
Fiſh round it, and the Liver all over the Head, ſtick
the Jaw-bones between, lay fried Parſley and Horſe-
radiſh and Barberryberries round the Diſh-edge, and
ſend it to Table.

To dreſs the Cod's Tail.

THE thick End of the Cod cut into Slices an
Inch thick, and lay them into an Earthen-diſh,
pour over them a Jill of Beer-vinegar, and ſtrew o-
ver ſome Salt; then take out the Bones, and cut the
Remainder into thin Slices for frying; ſeaſon with
Nutmeg,

Nutmeg, Pepper and Salt; then ſet on ſome Water in a broad Haſh-pan, and when it boils put in the Cod that is in the Vinegar; have no more Water then will cover it, and put in the Vinegar that it lay in; then dip the Cod out for frying, in Batter, made of half a Jill of ſtale Beer and Flour; if the Fiſh be for thoſe that abſtain from Fleſh, fry it in clarified Butter, if not, clean Fat; then take half a Hundred of Oyſters, and juſt plumb them; melt half a Pound of Butter, and put in the Oyſters, with a little of their Pickle, ſome Catchup, and a Spoonful of Muſhrooms; if you have a Double-diſh, fill it with hot Water; then take out your boiled Fiſh with a Fiſh-ſlice, and lay on the hot Diſh, pour over the Oyſter-ſauce, and lay the fry'd Fiſh all over: Lay Sippets, Barberry-berries, and Horſe-radiſh round, and ſend it up.

A Ragoo of Ling.

TAKE a Side of a Ling and cut a Quarter and a Half off the broad End, and cut a thick Slice off it, and a Piece of its Liver, and boil in Vinegar and Water; then take it up, and beat it in a Marble Mortar; add to it the Crumb of a *French* Roll; ſeaſon it with Nutmeg, Pepper and Salt, Thyme, Sweet-marjoram, and Parſley cut ſmall, a Glaſs of Rheniſh and an Egg, mix all well together with a Piece of Butter; take the Fiſh and cut off that Part next the Back, to make it of the ſame Thickneſs of the thinner Side, and take out the ſmall Bones; ſeaſon with Nutmeg, Pepper and Salt; beat two Yolks of Eggs in a Spoonful of Verjuice, and rub all over the Fiſh; then lay a thin Lair of the forced Fiſh on the Ling, and roll it tight up; roll a broad Tape round, butter an Earthen-diſh and lay it in, and ſet it into an Oven an Hour: Then fry a Pound of the Ling, cut thin into Collops, brown in Butter, and ſet on the Bones and Fins to boil in

a

a Sauce-pan, with an Anchovy, Horſe-radiſh, Shalot, Thyme, and Marjoram; when the Srength is
boiled out, ſtrain out the Broth into the Haſh-pan
to the fry'd Ling, and when it is ſtrong ſtrain it
through a Hair-ſieve; add to it half a Jill of pickled
Muſhrooms, a Spoonful of Cockles, twenty freſh
Oyſters, make twenty Balls of the forced Fiſh, and
fry in clarified Butter; then take the Fiſh out of
the Oven, pour off all its Gravy, ſtrain off the Fat,
and add to the Ragoo, thicken it with Butter-ſauce;
ſet the Collar in the Middle of the Diſh, and pour
over the Ragoo: Lay Sippets and fry'd Parſley
round the Diſh, and ſerve it up.

Scotch Collops *of* Ling.

CUT two Pound of Ling into Collops, and ſeaſon with *Jamaica* and Black-pepper, Nutmeg
and Salt; boil a Quarter of a Pound of Ling, and
take the Crumb of a *French* Roll, with a Slice of
very ſweet Butter and mix with it; add Thyme,
Sweet-marjoram, and Parſley cut ſmall, Nutmeg,
Pepper and Salt; work it all up together with an
Egg, and make them up into little Balls; then
make a Batter of half a Jill of Verjuice, the Yolks
of two Eggs, and a little Flour; dip each Collop
into the Batter, and fry them brown in clarified
Butter; take them into a Diſh, ſet them before the
Fire, and fry the Balls and lay by them; fry a Pound
of the Fiſh cut into thin Slices in Butter, put to it
a Pint of Fiſh-broth, an Anchovy, ſome Catchup,
and a Spoonful of Claret; when one Half is conſumed, ſtrain it off, and put it into a Sauce-pan, with
a little Butter and Flour, and boil it up; add to it
ſome Muſhrooms, and pickled Cockles: Lay the
fry'd Collops on a clean hot Diſh, the Balls all over
them, and pour over the Sauce; lay Sippets round
the Diſh, and garniſh with ſcraped Horſe-radiſh
and Barberry-berries, ſo ſerve it up.

A

A Brown Fricassey of Ling.

CUT out of the thick Part of the Ling a Pound and a Half, and cut into Collops as long as your Finger, as broad as Two, and the Thickness of a Beef-stake; season them with Mace, Cloves, Pepper and Salt; make a Batter of two Spoonfuls of White-wine Vinegar, two Yolks of Eggs, and a little Flour; dip the Fish in the Batter, and fry it in clarified Butter; cut the Liver after it is boiled and cold into thin Slices, and make a Batter of Vinegar and Flour, and dip each Slice of Liver in it, and fry it crisp; then have some strong Fish-gravy, made as before directed, and thicken it with Butter and Flour; add to the Gravy half a Jill of pickled Mushrooms, some Catchup and Claret, and boil it up: Lay the fry'd Fish in the Middle of the Dish, the fry'd Liver round by Way of Sippets, fry'd Parsley round the Dish-edge and some Barberry-berries; pour over the Sauce, and send it up hot.

A boiled Codling.

TAKE a Codling when it is in Perfection, which you may know by the ribby Shades on the Sides, and the Crease down the Back of the Head, or Sirkle more properly termed; rip it up and take out its Liver; turn the Tail of the Fish to its Head, and lay Salt all over it an Hour; have a Kettle or Pan a boiling, that will just hold it, so as to cover it with Water; take half of the Liver and shred it very small, boil it in a Sauce-pan in a Pint of Water with an Anchovy, let it boil to a Jill, strain it thro' a Hair-sieve into a Sauce-pan, and thicken it with Butter and Flour; take up your Fish, drain it, take off the Skin, and set it on a Dish: Garnish with green Parsley and Horse-radish, and send up your Sauce in a Bason.

A

A boiled Ling.

TAKE a Share of Ling, and boil it with the Liver, and put in some Salt with it into the Pan; take two Crabs, beat the Claws, and take out all the Meat; take some of the Body of the Crab, melt half a Pound of Butter, add to it the Meat of the Crabs, a little Black-pepper, and boil it; take up the Fish, laying it on a hot Dish, and send it up with the Skin on; slice the Liver and lay over it: Garnish with green Parsley, Horse-radish, and Barberry-berries.

To boil a Cod.

IF you can get a Cod hot out of the Sea, cut off the Head and Shoulders, and cut the Cod into Inch thick Slices, as much as will serve your Family, five Slices will make a substantial Dish; cut it as above directed, put it into an Earthen-pot, pour upon it a Pint of strong Beer Vinegar, and let it lie an Hour in the Vinegar, turning it over several Times; then have a Pan of Water boiling on a very good Fire, put in a Handful of Salt, and wash the Fish out of the Vinegar, pour it into the boiling Water and Salt, and let it boil fast half an Hour: For Sauce take thirty Oysters, and half a Pound of sweet Butter, melt it as Sauce; when the Oysters are clean washed, put them into the Butter and boil them up; add a Spoonful of Catchup and Spoonful of Mushrooms; take up the Fish and drain it over a hot Stove or Chafing-dish of hot Cinders a Minute or two; lay it on a hot Water-dish if you have one, otherwise let the Dish you lay it on be very hot, and pour over your Sauce: Garnish with Horse-radish, Parsley and Barberry-berries.

To

To *boil* Haddocks.

TAKE Haddocks when they are in Perfection, take out their Livers and Roes, and boil the Livers with the Haddocks, four will make a very good Diſh; take off their Heads, and skin them, cut them thro' the Middle, boil them, and broil their Roes before the Fire very well, they will take as much broiling as the Fiſh will boiling, *viz.* half an Hour; take them up, and place the Tails in the Middle of the Diſh, lay the other Halves between them, and lay their Livers and Roes all round the Diſh: Garniſh with green Parſley and Barberry-berries; and have for Sauce very ſweet Butter plain melted.

To *boil* Whitings.

WASH the Whitings clean, and with a ſharp Knife cut off all their Fins, skin them, take out their Eyes, and put each Tail through the Bone of the Head; boil as many as will do for your Purpoſe; for a Head-diſh or a Side-diſh: Garniſh with green Parſley; lay the Fiſh on a warm Diſh, and have plain melted Butter for Sauce.

To *fry* Whitings.

EITHER put them up as above directed, or cut off their Heads, rub them over with Yolks of Eggs, drudge Flour over them, and fry them in hot melted Fat, or clarified Butter; fry Parſley, ſet up their Tails in the Middle of the Diſh, and lay the fry'd Parſley round for garniſhing; lay ſome Barberry-berries over the Fiſh.

To *fry* Flounders.

TAKE Flounders or any Sort of Flat-fiſh, that is not over thick for frying, cut them on the Side of their Belly, and gut them, waſh them clean, and

and dry them with a coarse Cloth; take a sharp Case-knife and cut them cross and cross by Way of Diamond Cut; then rub them over with Yolks of Eggs, flour them, and fry them as above directed: Garnish with fry'd Parsley, and plain Butter-sauce; set up their Tails in the Middle of the Dish, and send them up to Table.

To *stew* Soles.

TAKE a Pair of Soles and skin them, fry them brown in Butter, take a Pint of strong Fish-gravy and put to them, add a little Mace, Nutmeg and Salt, let them stew over a slow Stove till there is no more Gravy than what is sufficient for Sauce; then add some pickled Mushrooms and a little melted Butter, lay Sippets round the Dish; then lay in your Soles, pour over your Sauce: Garnish with carved Lemon, and send them up.

To *crimp* Skate.

TAKE a Maiden Skate, and cut off all the bony Part, cut the two Wings into Pieces an Inch broad, and the Length of the Skate, wash it clean in Water, and let it lie in Vinegar and Salt an Hour; then have some Pump Water boiling on a hot Stove in a broad Hash-pan, into which put your Skate and a little of the Vinegar, and let it boil six Minutes; then take it up into a hot Dish, lay green Parsley round it; and have plain melted Butter-sauce, and send it up.

To *boil* Skate.

TAKE the broad Wing of a Maiden Skate and wash clean, hang it up on a Crook in the Air one Day; then boil it in Pump Water with Salt in it eight Minutes, take it up and take off the Skin,

and

and lay the two Wings on a Diſh whole: Garniſh
with green Parſley and Horſe-radiſh; have ſome
plain Butter-ſauce.

To ſtew Butts.

TAKE four Butts and waſh them clean, ſet them
on a Stove in a broad Haſh-pan, cover them
with Water, and put to them ſome Blades of Mace
and White-pepper tied up in a Muſlin-rag; then
take 30 freſh Oyſters, ſcald and beard them; when
the Fiſh is ſtewed, and the Gravy conſumed to no
more then what is required for Sauce, thicken it
with Butter and Flour; then put in your Oyſters,
and add a Spoonful of Rheniſh; lay Sippets and
Barberry-berries round the Diſh, ſet your Fiſh
Tails in the Middle, and ſend it up to the Table.

To boil Mackarel.

CUT your Mackarel in two, and if you have
three make a Star, ſet the Heads in the Middle,
and a Tail between each Head; boil them in a broad
Haſh-pan on a Stove in Salt and Water; have
Herbs, Parſley, and Fennel, boiled tender, and cut
very ſmall, and mix up with plain Butter melted:
Garniſh with green Parſley.

To ragoo Salmon.

TAKE a fore Jowl of Salmon, cut off the Head,
take out the Bone, and rub it all over with
Verjuice, or White-wine Vinegar; then boil the
Head, and take the Fiſh off it; grate Bread, with
a Slice of ſweet Butter, an Egg, green Thyme, Parſley, Sweet-marjoram cut very ſmall, Nutmeg,
Pepper, and Salt mix'd all together, and make Force-
meat; ſeaſon your Salmon with Nutmeg, Pepper,
and Salt, and put over the Inſide of it the Yolk of
an

an Egg; then lay on your Force-meat, roll it up, put it into a Pot, and ſet it into an Oven aſt Hour and a half; if it is not a Faſt-day, have half a Pint of good Gravy, a Quarter of a Pound of ſweet Butter, made for Sauce, and a Jill of ſcalded Gooſeberries; lay Sippets round the Diſh, and lay on your. Salmon: Garniſh with carved Lemon.

Scotch Collops *of* Salmon.

CUT out of a fore Jowl of Salmon Collops, rub each Collop with Verjuice, and ſeaſon with *Jamaica* and Black-pepper, Nutmeg, and Salt; make Force-meat and put it into a little round Baſon, and bake it in an Oven; then flour and fry the Collops; fry a Codling cut into Pieces, brown in Butter; add a Pint of Fiſh-broth, when it is ſtrong enough ſtrain it off, and thicken it with Butter and Flour; add to it a Jill of ſcalded Gooſeberries: Set the Force-meat in the Middle, lay the Collops round it, pour the Sauce all over it, and lay criſp Parſley round.

Olives *of* Salmon.

TAKE a hind Jowl of Salmon, skin and ſplit it, cut the firſt two half a Quarter in Length, and the Breadth of the Fiſh, and make the other End to the ſame Size; boil what Cuttings you leave for Force-meat, in the ſame Manner as is before directed; rub Yolks of Eggs all round each Piece of Fiſh, and ſeaſon it with Nutmeg, Pepper, and Salt; ſpread over each Collop a thin Lair of Force-meat, roll them up tight, lay them on a little long Tin-pan cloſe, and ſet them in an Oven half an Hour: For Sauce boil the Fiſh-bones, with an Anchovy, and Horſe-radiſh, and ſtrain it off; then add two Spoonfuls of Catchup, half a Jill of pickled Muſhrooms, thicken it with Butter and Flour, and lay the Olives: Garniſh with criſp Parſley.

To

To dress a Turbot.

BOIL the Head of a Turbot, save the Broth, and take off all the Fish; make Force-meat beat in a Mortar, adding Nutmeg, Pepper and Salt, two Eggs, grated Bread, and the Juice of a Lemon, mix a little of the Liver with the Force-meat, mix it all together, make it into Force-meat Balls, fry them in clarified Butter, and they will keep three Days; a Turbot of a moderate Size will be four very good Dishes, one boiled, and the Fins fry'd and laid round it, plain Butter-sauce, green Parsley, and scraped Horse-radish for garnishing; another Part ragoo'd, and the Fish-broth made Gravy by frying two or three Slices, and boiling in it; Force-meat Balls and Oysters made for the Ragoo, and the Turbot seasoned and broiled before the Fire, and set in the Middle of the Dish, and the Ragoo turn'd over it; Scotch Collops cut out of the thickest Part of the Turbot, dipp'd in Eggs and fry'd brown, after seasoning them with Nutmeg, Pepper and Salt; put on a Dish the Fish-gravy, Forced-balls, and pickled Mushrooms boiled, and pour over them Sippets and carved Lemon; a white Fricassey is, to cut out of the Turbot as many Pieces half Inch thick, and in Length two Inches, dip them in Whites of Eggs well beat, and fry them in clarified Butter; boil eight Yolks of Eggs, and take off the Beards of thirty Oyster, have white Fish-gravy, boil up the Oysters and thicken with melted Butter: Lay the Fricassey on the Dish, the Yolks round it, and pour over the Oysters and the Sauce.

To boil Salmon.

SCALE a Jowl of Salmon, make the Water very Salt, when it boils put in the Fish, and let it boil quickly; take Parsley, Fennel, and a little Mint

boil'd

boil'd and cut very ſmall, and lay round the Diſh-edge; pick and ſcald a Jill of Gooſeberries, and melt Butter: Lay your Salmon on a Diſh, and the Gooſe-berries all over it, and ſend up the Butter in a Sauce-boat.

To *bake* a Salmon.

TAKE a whole Salmon, take off its Skin, take out its Liver and Roe, and turn the Tail of the Fiſh to the Head, faſten it with Tape, cut the Fiſh a-croſs Diamond Shape, and rub it all over with Mace, Nutmeg, Pepper and Salt, Yolks of Eggs, and grated Bread; laying thin Slices of Butter all over the Back of the Salmon; then bake it two Hours in an Earthen-diſh; the Liver and Roe beat in a Mortar, add Nutmeg, Mace, Pepper, Salt, Thyme, Parſley, and Sweet-marjoram cut ſmall, and as much grated Bread as an Egg will make ſtiff enough to roll into Balls, and fry them; have Gravy made of Fleſh or Fiſh, into which put half a Jill of pickled Muſhrooms and the Force-balls: Set your Fiſh on a Diſh, lay Sippets and Lemon round, and pour on the Sauce.

To *ſtew* Tench.

PUT them alive into a Stew-pan, ſet them over a Stove till they are dead, let them be cloſe cover-ed; then take out the Tench, ſcale them, and take out their Guts, and let their Blood be in the Haſh-pan; then put in the Tench with a Pint of Water, a Jill of Claret, and let them ſtew till there is Sauce left to eat them, add nothing but Salt to it; lay Sippets and carved Lemon round the Diſh, and ſend it up.

To

To dreſs Pike.

TAKE a large Pike and ſcale him, take out his
Guts and Liver, boil and beat the Liver in a
Mortar; add to it a Slice of Butter, grated Bread,
Nutmeg, an Egg, Mace, Pepper, Salt, Thyme,
Sweet-marjoram, Parſley, and Chives cut ſmall; then
mix them well together, and put it into the Belly
of the Pike; then turn the Tail of the Pike to its
Head, and rub him all over with Yolk of Egg, and
ſtrew grated Bread upon the Egg; ſet him on a Tin
Dripping-pan before a clear Fire, and baſte it with
Butter, but take Care to turn it as it browns; when
it is thoroughly done, lay it on a warm Diſh: Gar-
niſh with criſp Parſley, and plain melted Butter for
Sauce, and ſend it to Table.

To ſtew Burn Trouts.

WASH as many Trouts as will make a ſubſtan-
tial Diſh, ſeaſon them with Pepper, Salt and
Nutmeg; lay them into a Pot that juſt holds them,
which muſt be of a longiſh Shape, and put to them
Butter and Shalot, and ſet them in an Oven two
Hours; then take them into a Stew-pan, and add
to them a Spoonful of Verjuice or the Juice of a
Lemon, and half a Jill of melted Butter; lay them
with their Tails in the Middle of your Diſh, and
their Heads round it: Garniſh with green Parſley.

To fry Trouts.

WASH and dry them with a Cloth, and dip
them in Vinegar and Flour, and fry them in
Butter ſo criſp, that they will ſtand round the Sauce-
baſon in the Diſh, with criſped Parſley round the
Diſh-edge, and ſend them up.

To fry Sparlings.

DON'T waſh them but dry them with a clean Cloth, and draw a ſmall Gut out of their Neck: Make Batter of Egg, Flour and Water, dip them in and fry them in clarified Butter, Hog's Lare, or Beef-fat; let it boil when you put in your Sparlings: For Sauce, plain melted Butter: Garniſh with fry'd Parſley and Barberry-berries.

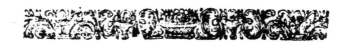

Inſtructions for potting FISH or FOWL.

To pot Salmon.

CUT a Salmon down the Middle, cut off the Head, ſcale and waſh it clean, take out the Chine-bone, and cut the Salmon to the Shape of your Pot or Pots; ſeaſon with Black-pepper and Salt; let your Pots be deep enough to contain a Double of the Salmon, and put into your Pot with it a Pound of Butter; bake it two Hours and take it out, pour off all the Gravy and Butter, and preſs it hard ſo as all may drain out of it; then ſet it into the Oven, and put the Butter into the Pot, but none of the Gravy, and let it ſtand four Hours longer in the Oven, in which Time all the Bones of the Salmon will be diſſolved to Fiſh; then take it out and drain off all the Butter, ſet a Preſs on the Salmon, and lay on a Weight to ſqueeze it well; when it is cold cover it with the Butter it was baked in, and ſome more Butter clarified.

To make Trouts *like potted* Jars.

TAKE black back'd Trouts that cuts Red, and wash very clean, and dry them with a Cloth; season them with Mace, Nutmeg, *Jamaica* and Black-pepper and Salt; put them into a Pot with Butter sufficient to boil them in, and set them in an Oven close covered; when they have been an Hour and a Half in the Oven, take them out, lay them on a flat Board, let all the Gravy drain from them, and take off all the Butter, but none of the Gravy: Then lay your Trouts into the Pot, and to every Lair add a little more of your Seasoning, according to what your Judgment supposes may be washed off in their boiling; put the Butter to them, and set them in an Oven three Hours and a Half, in which Time their Fins and Bones will become Fish; then take out your Pot, pour off the Butter they were baked in, and lay a small Weight on the Trouts; when they are cold, cover them with the Butter they were baked in; but if you have not enough to cover them with, clarify more Butter, and to have better than half an Inch Thickness above your Trouts.

To pot Lobsters.

TAKE large Lobsters when they are in their Prime, boil them, and take off their Claws and Tails; split the Tails, but keep the Claws as whole as you can, and take the Bone out of the Claws; season them with Black-pepper and Salt, and pot them, with plenty of Butter over them, and set them in an Oven an Hour; then take them out and drain all the Butter and Gravy off the Lobsters, take the Butter from the Gravy, and add as much clarified Butter as will cover the Lobsters: You must not press the Lobsters, but let the Butter run through them,

them, and when they are cut it will be a fine Mixture repreſenting of Marble.

To pot Lampar Eels.

TAKE Lampar Eels and cut off a Griſſel that lies down their Backs, skin and ſeaſon them with Mace, Nutmeg, Pepper and Salt, and put them cloſe into a Pot, with Butter over them and a Paper tied very cloſe, put them into an Oven two Hours; then draw off their Gravy and the Butter, ſqueeze out all the Gravy, and put the Butter into the Eels, and let them have four Hours more baking, in which Time their Bones will diſſolve; then take them out of the Oven, pour the Butter from them, and preſs the Eels cloſe down in the Pot; when they are cold cover them with the Butter they were baked in, adding more clarified Butter if wanted.——Theſe potted Eels are by moſt Judges thought to exceed all Sorts of potted Fiſh.

To pot Woodcocks.

PICK your Woodcocks clean, take out the Trail, and take off the Gizzard; work up ſome Pepper and Salt into half a Pound of Butter, and put the Size of a ſmall Chicken Egg into each Woodcock, put them into a Pot with their Breaſts turned down, lay as much Butter over as will cover them when it is melted, and ſet them two Hours in an Oven; then take out the Cocks, put out all the Butter and take it off the Gravy, put the Trails of the Woodcocks into their Gravy, ſet them into the Oven, and let them ſtew till it is thick; then put it all over the Cocks, put them cloſe down into the Pots, and cover them with the Butter they were baked in, adding more clarified Butter to them; let their Breaſts lie uppermoſt.

To pot Moor-fowl *or* Gore.

IF you have Plenty of Gore take out their Back-bones, and ſeaſon them with Black-pepper and Salt, cover them with Butter, lay their Breaſts down in the Pot, and ſet them two Hours and a Half in the Oven; when they are taken out have in Readi-neſs the Pots you deſign to pot them in, and take them out of the Pot they were baked in, turn their Breaſts up in the Pots, preſs them cloſe down, and cover them with clarified Butter.——Partridges and Pigeons much the ſame, only you are not to take the Back-bone off the Partridges or Pigeons, but let them be Pye Faſhion.

To pot a Hare.

SKIN it, and if not mangled, you need not waſh it, cut it into Joints, and ſeaſon with Mace, Nut-meg, *Jamaica* and Black-pepper, Salt, dried Thyme, Sweet-marjoram rubb'd ſmall and ſifted through a Hair-ſieve; put each Joint cloſe down into a Stew-ing-pot, with the Liver, Heart, and three Shalots, bake it till it is very tender: A young Hare will be tender in two Hours, an old one will take four Hours baking; when it is enough take it out, pour out all the Gravy and Butter into another Pot, ſtrip off all the Fleſh from the Bones, beat the Meat in a Wooden Bowl or Marble Mortar, and beat all the Butter that was taken from the Hare with the Meat, put it into Pots, and cover it with clarified Butter.

To pot Beef.

TAKE ſix Pounds of a Buttock of Beef and cut into Collops an Inch thick, beat an Ounce of Salt-petre to Powder, mix with four Ounces of Salt
and

and a little Sugar; lay a little of this on each Collop, and one Collop upon another, and put them into a Pot that juſt holds them; twenty-four Hours will make them red; then take them out and ſeaſon with *Jamaica* and Black-pepper, dried Thyme and Sweet-marjoram; put into it a Rocambole, and put it into a Stew-pan with the Marrow of three Beef-bones, or a Pound and a Half of Butter; when it is tender, take it out and beat it fine, and beat up with it the Marrow or Butter that it was baked with, or half of the Butter; put it into the Pots, cover with clarified Butter.

Potted Veal.

TAKE out of the Thick of a Leg of Veal with the Udder and Kell, and cut into Collops; ſeaſon with Mace, Nutmeg, Pepper and Salt, cover them cloſe into a Pot, and bake them two Hours; then take them out, and beat them with the Udder and Kell in a Mortar; when it is well mixed, put them into Pots, and cover with clarified Butter.

Potted Herrings.

WHEN Herrings are in Perfection, cut off their Heads, and take out their Roes and Back-bones, ſeaſon them with Black-pepper and Salt; roll each Herring up like a Collar round the Bottom of the Pot you are to bake them in, and ſet one Row upon another till your Pot is full; then tie a Paper cloſe about the Top of the Pot, and ſet them three Hours in an Oven; cover them over with Bay-leaves as ſoon as you draw them out, and fill the Pot as high as the Fiſh with White-wine Vinegar: Then put the Livers and Roes into a Pot by themſelves, and let them ſtand an Hour in the Oven, and then put the Roes into the Herrings: When they are diſh'd up, lay the Livers round the Herrings, and ſend up ſome of the Liquor: Have Fennel for garniſhing.

To

To collar Beef.

TAKE twenty Pounds of the Belly-end of the Flank of an Ox, and lay it in Salt and Water two Hours; then beat two Ounces of Saltpetre, mix it with a Pint of white Salt, and rub it all over the Beef, let it lie five Days, and turn it every Day; then waſh off all the Pickle, and dry it, ſpread it on a Board, cut it ſtraight, and lay the Cuttings a-croſs; ſeaſon with Nutmeg, Mace, Jamaica and Black-pepper, green Thyme, Sweet-marjoram, and Parſley cut ſmall; then lay your Cuttings croſs the Collar, roll it tight up with Tape, put it into a long Pot or Pan, and ſet it into an Oven all Night after the ſcorching Heat is off; in the Morning take it out, uncover it, take it out of the Pot, lay the Collar on a Tin, roll it round and preſs it; when cold take off the Tin, and keep it for Uſe.

To collar a Pig.

TAKE a good fat Pig, and after you have kill'd and dreſs'd it clean, waſh it well from the Blood, cut off the Head and ſplit it even in two, bone it, and waſh the Blood clean away; then dry the Fleſh well with Rubbers, laying it out at its full Length, and rubbing on it Yolk of Egg on the Inſide of each Half; ſeaſon with Nutmeg, Pepper, Salt, green Thyme, Sweet-marjoram, Parſley ſhred ſmall and ſtrew'd on, rolling each Side very tight, and tie a Cloth round each Side, and Tape upon the Cloth, and let it be tied cloſe at each End, and boil it two Hours; then take it up, undo the Sides, and tie it up again very tight: Make a Sauce of Bran-water and Salt, and a Jill of Vinegar, when it boils ſtrain it off, and when it is cold, put in the Pig, and keep for uſe.

To

To collar Ling.

TAKE the largeſt Ling you can get, cut it down the Middle, cut off all the Fins, and cut off the thick Part of it, to make it of an equal Thickneſs, cut it into three half Quarter lengths, and roll it up in as many Collars as will be of the Ling; make a ſtrong Brine of a Pound of Bay-ſalt and as much common Salt as will make an Egg ſwim to the Top; then ſet it on to boil, and boil the Liver of the Ling in the Brine; tie all the Collars firm with Tape, and boil them an Hour and a half; then take up the Collars, and ſtrain the Liquor into a deep Earthen-pot, and when it is cold, put in the Collars: It eats like Sturgeon, and is eaten with Muſtard, Vinegar, Oil and Sugar.

To marble a Calf's Head.

TAKE a large fat Calf's Head, waſh it through many Waters, take out the Eyes, and boil it till all the Bones will come out from the Fleſh; then have for Seaſoning, Mace, Nutmeg, Pepper, Salt, green Thyme, Sweet-marjoram and Parſley cut ſmall; take out all the Bones and the Skin of the Palate, cut the Head on a Shreading-board, and put it into a Cloth when it is very hot, and tie it up cloſe: It will cut out like Marble, and is a pretty Diſh for a ſecond Courſe.

To collar Calves Feet.

TAKE a Gang of good Feet, and boil them in ſoft Water as for Gelly, take out the Feet, and make great Haſte to take out all the Bones while the Feet is hot; then cut and throw a little Salt over them, and put them cloſe down in a Pint Water-glaſs, and carve it in cutting like Brawn, in thin

Slices;

Slices; when you take it out of the Glaſs, lay the carved Slices round, and ſet the Collar in the Middle of the Diſh: Garniſh with green Parſley.

To make a Veal Soop.

TAKE a Leg of Veal, cut off the Fleſh, break the Bones, and put Bones and Meat into a Stewing-pan, add to it two Quarts of Water, ſtick ſix Cloves in a large Onion, two Carrots, two Turnips and a little Salt; cover it very cloſe, paſte down the Lid, and ſet it all Night in an Oven; take it out in the Morning, pour off all your Soop, ſkim off the Fat, and put the Soop into a clean Flannel-bag, uſed for nothing but ſtraining Gravy, and put it into a very clean Haſh-pan; add to it an Ounce of Vermicelli, and let it boil gently; grate half an Ounce of Loaf-ſugar all over the Bottom of the Haſh-pan, and ſet it on ſome clear Cinders till the Sugar boils and turns to the Colour of Treacle; then put to it a little of the Soop, and boil till all the Colour is mixt with the Soop; then mix it with the other Soop; toaſt two thin Slices of Bread cut into Dices, and put into the Soop-diſh, lay boiled Rice round the Diſh-edge, and pour in the Soop; or ſend it up a Canteen. The Veal will be very good to eat cold, minced or potted, with adding Seaſoning to it, as directed for potted Veal.

A Sellery Soop.

IF you would go to the thrifty Way of Soop making, boil a Leg of Mutton for a Family Diſh, ſtrain your Broth into an Earthen-pot, and let it ſtand all Night; take off the Top, pour off the Clear, and ſtrain the Bottom through your Flannel-bag; take four Pounds of the Buttock of an Ox, and put your Broth into a ſmall Boiler; put in your Beef, and be careful to ſkim it when it begins

to boil; when you have skim'd it well, waſh as
much Sellery and cut it, as will fill a Pint-baſon;
after the Sellery has ſtewed with the Beef three
Hours, add a Pint-baſon of diced Turnips and Carrots of each an equal Quanity, and let it ſtew an
Hour; then boil Spinage and lay round the Diſh-
edge, toaſt Bread and cut into Sippets: Set the Beef
in the Middle of the Diſh, pour in the Soop, lay
the Sippets round, and ſend it up.

A Cabbage Soop.

TAKE four Quarts of Beef, Mutton, or Veal-
broth, and put into a ſmall Boiler, and ſix
Pounds of the beſt Part of the Beef without Bones,
put the Beef into the Pot, let it boil, and skim it
well; then take a White-cabbage and cut it into
four Quarters, cut out the Core, and put it to the
Beef; let it ſtew four Hours, keeping it cloſe covered, and be ſure to let it ſtew very gently; then
ſet the Beef in the Middle of the Diſh, lay the Cabbage round it, and pour over the Soop: The Beef
and Cabbage is as good as the Soop.

To make a Soop without Water.

TAKE a Stone of Beef, a Stone of Mutton, a
Stone of Veal, and cut all into Inch thick
Collops; then take a large Earthen-pot, lay in a
Lair of Collops and a Lair of ſliced Turnips, then
Collops and ſliced Carrots, cover that with Fleſh;
then have Sellery, and intermix the Meat with the
Roots and Sellery; when all is put into the Pot
cover it cloſe, ſet it into a hot Oven, and let it
ſtand two Hours; then take it out, pour off all your
Gravy, and ſtrain it through a Flannel-bag, and ſet
it another Hour into the Oven; then drain off all
your Gravy, and filter it through a Flannel-bag into
your

your other Soop: Put it into a clean Haſh-pan, and add to it an Ounce of Vermicelli, boil it ten Minutes; then cut ſome Bread and toaſt brown, and put a little into the Soop-diſh, pour in the Soop, and ſend it up.

To make a white Soop.

BOIL a Neck of Veal to Rags, ſtick ſix Cloves in an Onion, and boil it all the Time the Meat boils; then ſtrain it off, and skim off all the Fat, filter it through a Flannel-bag, and put it into a clean Haſh-pan; add to it half a Pound of Rice, and let it boil ſoftly Half an Hour; take a Quarter of a Pound of Rice, and let it boil a Quarter of an Hour in fair Water, and put it into a Hair-ſieve to let the Water run from it; then take a Pennyworth of Saffron, infuſe it in two Spoonfuls of Water, put the Rice into it, and it will make it yellow; then put a Rim of Paſte round the Brim of the Diſh, lay the Rice round the Edge of the Diſh; then boil up the Soop, and take the Crumb of a *French* Roll, raſp it, and ſet it in the Middle of the Diſh; pour on the Soop, and ſend it up.

To make a Hodge-podge.

TAKE a Neck of Mutton, cut it into Chops, and put a Gallon of Water to it, and as it begins to boil skim it well; add to it two Ounces of Pearl-barley, two Turnips, two Carrots, cut into Dices, a Pint of green Peaſe, green Thyme, Sweet-marjoram, Parſley, and two Cabbage Lettices cut ſmall, ſome Chives, and let all boil together, till there is as much as will fill a good Diſh, and ſo ſend it up.

To make a Portable Soop.

TAKE a Buttock of Ox Beef and cut into Inch thick Collops; take three Carrots and cut into Slices, and slice four Turnips, and cut as much Sellery as will fill a Quart; then lay into your Pot a Lair of Beef, lay Roots and Sellery upon it, and so intermix the Beef, Roots, Sellery and all close together down in an Earthen-pot that just holds it; then cover and paste the Pot, and set it in an Oven three Hours; then take it out, strain off all the Fat and let the Gravy run through a Flannel-bag; then put it into a Stew-pan, set it on a clear Stove, let it boil till it is thick, and stirring it with a Spoon; when it begins to stick take it off, put it into Tea-cups, let it stand till it is cold, turn it into a clean Linen-cloth, turn them once a Day into a dry Part, and set it in the Sun now and then till it is perfectly dry. This is for a Travelling Soop; an Ounce of this when it is dry will make a Porringer of Soop, cut it and put it into a Sauce-pan, and add Water to it, set it on the Fire and it will dissolve; toast some Bread, cut it into Dices, and pour in the Soop.

A Pease Soop.

TAKE two Quarts of Marrow Pease, put to them two Gallons of Water, let them boil till one Half is consumed and the Pease burst; take a Sieve and strain your Pease, putting some of the Pulp through the Sieve; then set it on a Stove in a Hash-pan, cut some Sellery and boil with it, rub dry Mint and sift it through a Sieve; mix with the Soop some *Jamaica* Pepper powder'd, and two Anchovies; cut some Bread into Dices and fry brown, and put into your Soop-dish; when the Soop is boiled to two Quarts, put to it a Slice of Butter

and

and half a Jill of thick sweet Cream; just as it boils put it into your Soop-dish, and send it up.

A green Pease Soop.

TAKE two Quarts of old green Pease, put them into a Gallon of Water, and let them boil till they are consumed to two Quarts; then strain them through a Hair-sieve, and put through all the Pulp you can get into a Hash-pan; dry some green Mint, put it through a Sieve, and add to it, with some powdered *Jamaica* Pepper, an Anchovy, and a Jill of young green Pease; let the Soop on a Stove, and let it boil gently half an Hour: Then take some of the Husks of the Pease and some young Spinage, beat them in a Mortar, squeeze the Juice into the Soop, and let it boil up; add a Slice of sweet Butter, half a Jill of Cream, and fry'd Bread cut into Dices, put them into the Dish, pour in the Soop, and send it up.

To make a Cheshire Cheese Soop.

PUT the Crumb of a Penny-loaf into three Pints of Water, boil it, and grate half a Pound of old *Cheshire*, put it into the Bread and boil it.

To make an Onion Soop.

TAKE a Quart of green Pease, put three Quarts of Water to it, and let it boil to two Quarts; then take six Onions, two Cabbage Lettices, green Thyme, Sweet-marjoram, Parsley, green Mint and Chives all cut small; take a Quarter of a Pound of Butter into a Frying-pan, make it hot, put in the Onions and Herbs, fry them, and put into the Soop; add a little Black-pepper and Salt to your Taste, cut a large Slice of Bread, and toast it brown; pour the Soop into the Dish, and cut the Bread into Dices, pour over the Soop, and send it up.

To

To make a Turnip Soop.

BOIL a Pennyworth of Turnips and Carrots in ſix Quarts of Water and a Pennyworth of Sellery, let them boil into three Quarts and ſtrain it off; then cut the Turnips and one Carrot into Dices, and cut the Tops of half a Hundred of Aſparagus very ſmall; take a Piece of Butter into a Frying-pan, and make it hot, fry the Carrots, Turnips, and Aſparagus, and put them into the Soop; add a Quarter of a Pound of Pearl-barley, and ſalt it to your Taſte, duſt in a little Pepper, and ſend it up.

To make a Fiſh Soop.

BOIL a large Tail of Cod or Ling with a good Quantity of Haddocks Heads, fry ſome ſplit Haddocks brown in Butter, and when the Fiſh-broth is ſtrong ſtrain it into the fry'd Haddocks; then let it boil, and ſtrain it off when you judge it ſtrong enough, skim off all the Fat, and put the Broth into a clean Haſh-pan; add to it two Ounces of Sagoe, and let it boil, ſtick eight Cloves into two large Onions and add to the Soop; skin a Whiting and put its Tail through its Head, rub it with the Yolk of Egg, fry it in clarified Butter, and ſet it in the Middle of the Soop-diſh; ſcald half a Hundred of Oyſters in their own Liquor, take off all their Beards, and put them into your Soop-diſh: Lay Shrimps round the Diſh-edge, pour your Soop upon the Oyſters, ſet the Whiting in the Middle, and ſend it up.

To make a Craw Fiſh Soop.

TAKE four Codlings and cut into Slices, ſeaſon them with Pepper and Salt, and put them into an Earthen-pot, add to them a Bundle of ſweet
Herbs

Herbs, some Shalots, and two Quarts of Water,
cover the Pot close, paste it down, and let it stand
three Hours in an Oven; in the mean Time take a
hundred Craw-fish out of their Shells after they are
boiled, beat ten of them and as many Shrimps in a
Mortar, grate the Crumb of a *French* Roll, a Slice
of Butter, an Egg, green Thyme, Sweet-marjoram,
Parsley, Chives, Nutmeg, Pepper and Salt; mix
all these well together, make up into little Balls, and
brown them before the Fire, or set them in an Earthen-plate into an Oven; when your Fish has been
the above Time in the Oven, take it out, and pour
it into a Flannel-bag, let it run into a Hash-pan, and
set it on a Stove; cut the Craw-fish small and add
to it, pick the Meat out of the Claws of the Crabs
and lay round the Edge of the Soop-dish: Toast
Bread and cut it into Dices, pour the Soop into the
Dish, put the forced Balls and toasted Bread all over
it, and send it up.

A Calf Foot Soop.

TAKE the Stock that is boiled of a Gang of
Calf's Feet, as if for Gellies, and when it is cold
take off the Top and Bottom, put the other into a
Hash-pan, set it on a slow Stove, and put to it a
Stick of Cinnamon; take a Quarter of a Pound of
Rice, boil it in Water a Quarter of an Hour, and
put it into a Sieve to let the Water run from it;
then take the Yolks of six Eggs and the Whites of
two, and beat them well in a Bason; then put three
Jills of thick Cream to the Soop, and sweeten it to
your Taste, lay Rice round the Edge of the Soop-
dish, and put what remains into the Soop; then
take a Pint of White-wine and mix with the Eggs,
grate in a little Nutmeg and mix all with the Soop,
tossing it up with a Whisk, and stir it on the Stove
till it is very near boiling, but by no Means let it
boil, for that will break it; it must be smooth and

S   thick,

thick, pour it into the Diſh, and ſend it up.—The Receipt of this Soop was deſired of me by three Baronets Ladies: It is a very good Supper Soop.

An Orange Pudding.

BOIL two *Seville* Oranges in ſeveral Waters till they are tender, take out all the In-meat, and beat the Skins to a Paſte in a Mortar; add to it half a Pound of fine Powder-ſugar, half a Pound of Butter beat to Cream in a Mortar; then take out the Seed and the Strings, and add the Pulp of the Oranges to it, and the Yolks of ten Eggs, beat all together till it is ſmooth; then lay a Sheet of Puff-paſte all over your Diſh, pour in your Pudding and bake it three Quarters of an Hour.

A boiled Orange Pudding.

GRATE the Rind of two *Seville* Oranges, and beat it in a Mortar to a Paſte; put a Quarter of a Pound of Naple Biſcuits into a Pint of thick Cream, mix this with the Paſte of Orange, and ſweeten it to your Taſte; beat up five Eggs, mix all well together, flour a Pudding-cloth, put in your Pudding, and put it into a Pot of boiling Water, an Hour will boil it: Take White-wine, a little Sugar and ſweet melted Butter for Sauce.

A Lemon Pudding.

PARE the Skin off three Lemons, and boil them in ſeveral Waters till they are tender; then beat them in a Mortar till they become Paſte; add half a Pound of Butter and half a Pound of Sugar, beat all ſmooth; take eight Eggs, leave out the Whites of four, and add a Glaſs of Rheniſh-wine; lay a very thin Sheet of Puff-paſte over the Diſh, and pour on
the

the Pudding: Three Quarters of an Hour will bake it.

A boiled Lemon Pudding.

GRATE off the yellow Rind of three Lemons, and beat it into a Paſte in a marble Mortar; take the Crumb of a three Half-penny *French* Roll, boil a Pint of thick Cream and pour upon it, ſweeten it to your Taſte, beat five Eggs and mix with it; flour a Cloth well and put in your Pudding: After all is well mixt, an Hour will boil it, and have for Sauce plain melted Butter, Sugar, the Juice of a Lemon, a little White-wine, and grate Loaf-ſugar all over the Diſh.

A Sego Pudding.

BOIL three Ounces of Sego in a Quart of Water a Quarter of an Hour, put it into a Hair-ſieve, and drain out all the Water; take a Quart of Cream and boil the Sego in it till it is thick, ſet it to cool, and ſweeten it to your Taſte; then beat eight Eggs, the Whites of Four leave out, let them be well beat, and mix with the Pudding, grate into it a little Nutmeg, and lay a Sheet of Puff-paſte over a Diſh, and pour in your Pudding; an Hour will bake it.

A Carrot Pudding.

TAKE half a Pound of boiled Carrots and beat to Paſte in a Mortar, add a Quarter of a Pound of Sugar, grate a little Nutmeg, melt a Quarter of a Pound of Butter, beat five Eggs and mix all well together; lay Puff-paſte over the Diſh, pour in the Pudding, and bake it half an Hour.

A.

A boiled Carrot Pudding.

TAKE half a Pound of boiled Carrots and beat in a Mortar to Paste; take the Crumb of a *French* Roll and foak in thick Cream, beat eight Eggs, and leave the Whites of Four out; mix all well with the Carrots, and grate in a little Nutmeg, rub a Piece of Butter on your Pudding-cloth, and pour on the Pudding, tie it faft and boil it an Hour; grate Sugar all over the Difh, and let your Sauce be plain Butter, Sugar, and a little White-wine; turn the Pudding into the Difh, and pour on your Sauce.

An Apple Pudding.

TAKE half a Pound of pared and cored Apples, boil them ten Minutes in Water, beat them in a Mortar to Pulp, and fweeten to your Tafte; then melt a good Slice of Butter and mix with the Pulp; take the Yolks of eight Eggs beat well, and a little grated Lemon-peal; mix all well together, and lay Puff-pafte over a Difh, pour in the Pudding, and bake it half an Hour.

A Rice Pudding.

TAKE three Ounces of the Flour of Rice and three Jills of new Milk, and put it into a Brafs-pan over a clear Fire, ftirring it with a Spoon all the Time; when it boils take it off, and ftir in a Slice of Butter, grate in fome Nutmeg, and fweeten to your Tafte, beat up fix Eggs and leave out three Whites; mix all well together, and lay Puff-pafte over the Difh, pour in your Pudding, and bake it half an Hour.

A

A *boiled* Rice Pudding.

TAKE half a Pound of Rice and boil it half an Hour in Water, put it into a Hair-sieve, and let the Water drain from it; then beat up the Yolks of eight Eggs, with a Jill of sweet Cream, grate some Nutmeg, and mix all with the boiled Rice, butter a Cloth, put in the Pudding and boil it an Hour; grate Sugar all over the Edge of the Dish, and for Sauce have Butter, Sugar and White-wine; set the Pudding on its Dish, and send up your Sauce in a Bason.

A Hunter's Pudding.

TAKE a Pound of Flour, a Pound of Currants, and a Pound of Beef-suet, pick and wash the Currants clean, shred the Suet very small, and mix all together; beat up six Eggs with a Jill of Cream, grate in Nutmeg, and mix all well together; flour a Cloth, and boil it two Hours and a Half: For Sauce, Butter and Sugar.

A Bread *and* Butter Pudding.

TAKE a Penny *French* Roll two Days old, cut off all the Crust, and cut the Crumb into thin Slices, spreading it as you cut it very thin with Butter on each Slice; then take a Quarter of a Pound of Rasins stoned, half a Pound of Currants well washed and pick'd; then lay a Lair of Bread and Butter, and upon that Fruit in a Pudding-dish, so cover the Fruit with the buttered Bread, and when it is disposed of into your Dish, beat up five Eggs with a Quart of new Milk, sweeten it to your Taste, and put to it a Glass of Rose-water, pour it into the Dish upon the Bread and Fruit, and bake it an Hour.

A boiled Bread Pudding.

TAKE a Pound of the Crumbs of *French* Rolls, boil a Pint of new Milk and pour upon it; take the Yolks of ſeven Eggs, and the Whites of Three, beat very well, and mix with the Milk and Bread; grate in a little Nutmeg, butter your Cloth, pour in your Pudding, tie it up tight, and boil it an Hour: For Sauce plain Butter.

A boiled Cuſtard Pudding.

TAKE a Quart of Cream and boil with ſix Laurel-leaves; ſet it to cool and break fourteen Eggs, leave out the Whites of five, and beat them very well; ſweeten to your Taſte, put in your Sugar when the Cream is on the Fire that it may diſſolve and mix with the Cream; then when it is cold mix the Eggs with it, have a very fine Cloth to boil it in, rub ſome Butter on your Cloth, put on your Pudding, tie it tight, put it into boiling Water, and let it boil an Hour; grate Sugar all over the Diſh, turn in the Pudding, and ſend it up.

To make a Calf's Feet Pudding.

TAKE half a Pound of Calf's Feet-meat after it is boiled tender, and all the Bones ſeparated from the Meat, blanch half a Pound of *Jourdon* Almonds, and ſhred the Calf's Feet and Almonds as ſmall as poſſible; pick and waſh half a Pound of Currants, and mix with the Feet; add a little Sugar, and a little grated Nutmeg; beat up the Yolks of eight Eggs in a Jill of thick Cream, mix all well together, lay Puff-paſte all over a Diſh, put on the Pudding, and ſend it to the Oven: Half an Hour will bake it.

A

A boiled Calf's Feet Pudding.

TAKE half a Pound of Calf's Feet, and half a Pound of Beef-fuet and fhred very fmall; half a Pound of pick'd Currants, a Quarter of a Pound of Rafins, and mix all together; foak the Crumb of a Penny Loaf in new Milk, break five Eggs and beat and mix all well together; butter a Cloth, put on your Pudding, boil it an Hour and a half, grate Sugar all over the Difh, and turn on your Pudding: Have for Sauce Butter and Sugar, pour it over the Pudding, and fend it up.

To make an Almond Pudding.

BLANCH half a Pound of *Jourdon* Almonds, and beat them in a Marble Mortar to Pafte; take three Jills of thick fweet Cream, and fweeten to your Tafte; add to it two Pennyworth of Orange Flower-water; take feven Eggs leaving out the Whites of Four, and mix all together; laying Puff-pafte over the Difh, pour on your Pudding, and bake it in an Oven three Quarters of an Hour.

A Goofeberry Pudding.

TAKE half a Pound of Butter, break into it a Pound of Flour, and rub it fmall; beat two Yolks of Eggs in a Jill of Water, take as much of this as you need to work the Butter and Flour into a Pafte, roll it into a Sheet, let it be thin round the Edge, put in a Quart of Goofeberries, and near a Quarter of a Pound of Powder-fugar; then rub it round the Edge of the Pafte with Water, gather it up together clofe, put it into a Pudding-cloth, tie it and boil it an Hour: For Sauce plain Butter and Sugar.

A

A Prune Pudding.

TAKE a Pound and a half of Flour, and a Pint of new Milk and mix it with; beat fix Eggs and mix with the Milk and Flour; then take a Pound of Prunes, half a Pound of ſtoned Raſins, and half a Pound of Currants, mix all with the Flour and Milk, and let it boil three Hours: For Sauce have plain melted Butter and Sugar, and a little Roſe-water; grate Sugar all over the Diſh, turn on the Pudding, and ſo ſend it to Table.

A Marrow Pudding.

TAKE half a Pound of Marrow and cut very ſmall, three Quarters of a Pound of Flour, half a Pound of ſtoned Raſins, and half a Pound of well picked Currants, mix all well together, with five Eggs, a Jill of Cream, and grate in ſome Nutmeg; put the Pudding in a Cloth, and boil it two Hours, grate Sugar over the Diſh, and have Sweet-ſauce.

A French Bean Pudding.

TAKE a Quart of young *French* Beans, boil and blanch them, and beat them in a Mortar to a fine Paſte; add to the Glaſs of Verjuice, a Quarter of a Pound of Powder-ſugar, half a Pound of Butter, and ſeven Eggs, the Whites of Three left out, beat all well together; lay a Puff-paſte on the Diſh, pour on the Pudding, and bake it three Quarters of an Hour: For Sauce have melted Butter, White-wine and Sugar.

A Ratafia Pudding.

TAKE a Quart of ſweet Cream, and boil fix Laurel-leaves two Minutes, take them out, and let the Cream ſtand till it be cold; then take
half

half a Pound of Flour and mix with the Cream, and beat ſix Eggs and mix all together; add a little Salt, butter your Pudding-cloth, pour in the Pudding, tie it tight, and boil it an Hour and a half; grate Sugar all over the Diſh, have Sweet-ſauce, turn in your Pudding, and ſend it up.

A Tanſy Pudding.

GRATE the Crumbs of two Penny *French* Rolls, beat up eight Eggs with a Pint of Cream, and mix the Bread with it; then take a Handful of Tanſy, and a Handful of Spinage, and beat in a Mortar, ſqueeze the Juice through a Sieve into the Pudding, and ſweeten to your Taſte; take a Quarter of a Pound of Butter into a Frying-pan, pour your Tanſy into the Pan, ſet it over a clear Fire or Stove, and ſtir it all the Time till it is thick; then put it into a Diſh and let it ſtand half an Hour in an Oven; then cut a *Seville* Orange into eight Parts, and ſet round the Diſh: Have for Sauce White-wine and Sugar.

A Gelly Tanſy.

TAKE a Quart of ſweet Cream, and the Yolks of twelve Eggs, and ſweeten to your Taſte; take a Handful of Tanſy, and a Handful of green Wheat and beat in a Mortar, ſqueeze the Juice through a Hair-ſieve, put it to the Cream and Yolks of Eggs, mix it well together, and ſet it ten Minutes in a ſlow Oven: Garniſh with Orange.

An Herby Pudding.

TAKE a Pint of Groats and boil half an Hour in Water, and put them into a Sieve to drain the Water from them; then take green Thyme, Parſley, Sweet-marjoram, Pot-marjoram, Dates and
young

young Onions of each an equal Quantity, cut them very small and mix with the Groats; then take a Jill of thick Cream, and the Yolks of ten Eggs, and mix all well together with a little Salt; then butter a Cloth and tie it in, and boil it an Hour: Have plain Butter for Sauce.

A Liver Pudding.

TAKE the Liver of a good Calf and cut one half into Inch thick Slices; take a Quart of Water into a broad Hash-pan, set it on a hot Stove, when it boils put in the sliced Liver, and let it boil five Minutes; then take it up and cut it very small on a Shreding-board; take half the Weight of the Liver of Beef-suet and mix with it; add green Thyme, Parsley, Sweet-marjoram, Chives cut small, Nutmeg, Pepper and Salt, and beat six Eggs and mix with it; put it into a Pudding-cloth, and boil it three Quarters of an Hour: For Sauce have Gravy and Butter.

Apple Dumplins.

TAKE large Apples pare and core them, make a cold Paste, and roll out a Sheet for each Apple; cut a Lemon-skin very small, and put a little into the Middle of each four Quarters of the Apple, but no Sugar, it may be sweetened at the Table as People like; roll up one Apple in every Sheet of Paste, take Care to leave no Room for the Water to enter in, and boil them three Quarters of an Hour; have Butter and Sugar to eat the Dumplins with.

To make Spice Dumplins.

TAKE a Quarter of a Pound of Butter and a Jill of Cream, and boil together, work it up with Flour; add to it some Cinnamon beat fine, and grate

in

in ſome Nutmeg, a Quarter of a Pound of ſton'd Raſins, and ſome Currants, make them into little Dumplins and fry them; then grate Sugar over them: For Sauce, have plain melted Butter and Sugar.

An Amalet *of* Eggs.

TAKE twelve Eggs and beat well, boil half a Hundred of Aſparagus, and cut the green Ends ſmall, and mix with the Eggs; then make ſome clarified Butter hot in a Frying-pan on a Stove or clear Fire, into which put the Eggs and Graſs caſt over them, a little Pepper and Salt, and fry them a nice brown; the Amalet will be an Inch thick; lay it on a Diſh, and garniſh with Parſley: Have Vinegar and Butter for Sauce.

Clary Pancakes.

MAKE a Batter of a Jill of Cream, four Eggs, and four Spoonfuls of Flour, a Glaſs of Sack, grate a little Nutmeg, and beat all well together; take a large Leaf of Clary and waſh it clean, take ſome clarified Butter into a Frying-pan, and pour in Half of your Batter, and lay on your Clary Leaf, cover it with the other Half of your Batter, and fry it very criſp on both Sides: Have Sugar and hot White-wine for Sauce, and grate Sugar round the Diſh.

Wafer Pancakes.

TAKE a Pint of Cream, three Spoonfuls of Flour, and five Eggs; then put a Slice of Butter into a Piece of thin Linen-cloth; take a Girdle and ſet on a clear Fire, rub the butter'd Cloth over the Bottom of it, and pour on a large Spoonful of Batter, ſo fry them very quick and criſp.

Rataſia

Ratafia Pancakes.

BOIL ſix Laurel-leaves in a Pint of Milk, take them out and ſet the Milk to cool; then beat up four Eggs with a little of the Milk and Flour, and add the Remainder of the Milk, let the Batter be thin, and take a Frying-pan, put into it a Slice of Butter and let it be hot, and pour in your Batter, but not to make your Pancakes thick; fry them criſp, and ſend them ſingle to the Table hot.

Apple Fritters.

MAKE a Batter of a Jill of Cream, Flour, and four Eggs, let it be thick and beat it half an Hour; add to it a Glaſs of Orange-flower Water, grate in a little Nutmeg, and Cinnamon finely beat and ſifted, and ſweeten it with Loaf-ſugar; cut off the Skins of ſome large Pippins, and cut round Slices off them, taking out the Seeds; then take a Pint of clarified Butter or Hog's Lare into a little Haſh-pan, and ſet it over a clear Stove; when it is hot dip each ſliced Apple into the Batter, and boil it up, turning each Fritter, and they will be as round as Balls; grate Sugar over them, and ſend them up.

To fry Cream.

TAKE a Pint of Cream and ſweeten it to your Taſte, grate in ſome Nutmeg and mix with it; cut a large Slice round a Six-penny Loaf an Inch thick and ſquare, lay it on a clean Board and pour on the Cream by degrees, ſo as to let the Bread ſoak moſt of it up, and have ſome clarified Butter in a Frying-pan upon a clear Stove or Fire; let the Butter be hot, and with a Knife cut the Bread into Inch ſquare Dices; fry them criſp in the clarified Butter,

and

and put them on a Diſh, grate Sugar all over them, and ſend them up.

A Calf Foot Gelly.

FIRST ſcald a Gang of Calf Feet, ſcrape off all the Hair very clean, and take off the Hoofs; have a very clean Pot with two Gallons of ſoft Water, put in your Feet, and let them boil ſoftly till there is three Quarts; then ſtrain it into an Earthen-pot, let it ſtand till it is cold and take all the Fat off the Top, put the Stock into a clean Pan, beat the Whites of eight Eggs to a Froth and add to it, with the Juice of three Lemons and the Skin of one, three Quarters of a Pound of ſingle refin'd Sugar, and mix all well together with a Pint of Rheniſh-wine; ſet the Pan on a Stove or clear Fire, and have a clean Flannel-bag ready to run it through; when it boils pour it into the Bag, and let it run into a Baſon, put it into the Bag again till it runs off very clear, then you may glaſs it or put it in Baſons; when it is cold you may get three Laurel-leaves, lay them upon the Top of the Baſon, and with your Finger looſen the Gelly from the Side, whelm a Diſh on the Baſon, turn the Gelly upſide down, and it makes a pretty Globe.

To make Hartſhorn Gelly.

TAKE half a Pound of Hartſhorn Shavings and put into a Pan with two Quarts of Water, and let it boil till one half is conſumed; then ſtrain it off and take the Whites of five Eggs beat to a Froth, a Quarter of a Pound of Sugar, a Jill of Rheniſh, the Juice of a Lemon, and a Stick of Cinnamon, mix all well together and ſet on the Fire; when it boils ſtrain it through a Flannel-bag as above directed.

To *make* Calf Foot Flummery.

TAKE the Stock of a Gang of Calf's Feet, after they are boiled and cool'd, and the Top taken off and the Bottom left; let your Pan be clean, and put in this Stock into a clean Pan, beat a Quarter of a Pound of bitter Almonds and put to it, and ſweeten to your Taſte, and let it boil half an Hour; then take a Pint of Cream and add to it, and ſtrain it through a clean Linen-cloth into a Delf-bowl, and keep it ſtirring till it is almoſt cold; then put it into Shapes of various Forms, ſuch as Scallops, Shells, Harts, &c. After you have ſet them to Gelly, when you want them for Uſe, you muſt preſs them round with your Fingers which will looſen them, and make them turn out ſmooth and eaſy on your Diſhes.

To *make* Hartſhorn Flummery.

TAKE Half a Pound of the Shavings of Hartſ-horn, two Ounces of Iſing-glaſs, and three Quarts of Water boiled to three Pints over a ſlow Fire, ſtrain it through a Gelly-bag, and put it into a clean Pan again, and ſet it on a clear Fire; add to it a Stick of Cinnamon, and let it boil to a Quart, and ſweeten to your Taſte; then put to it a little Orange-flower Water and a Jill of Cream, and ſtrain it off through a Linen-cloth, and ſtir it till it is al-moſt cold: Then put it into ſundry Shapes as above directed.

To *make* Leach.

BOIL the Stock of Calf's Feet as ſtrong as for Flummery, and clear them with the Whites of Eggs, Lemon-juice, White-wine, Sugar, and powder two Penny-worth of Cocheneal, and boil with it;
ſtrain

ſtrain it through a Gelly-bag, and put it into Flummery Shapes.

Steeple Cream.

BEAT and sift through a Hair-seive a Pound of double refin'd Sugar; and take a Quarter of a Pound of Currant-gelly, and the Whites of two Eggs into a China of Delf-bowl, and beat it an Hour with a Silver-spoon: It is a pretty Side-dish.

Raſp Cream.

TAKE a Quart of Cream, a Quarter of a Pound of Raſp-juice, mix the Cream with the Raſp-juice, and put it into a China-bowl; take a Chocolate-ſtick and mill up the Cream as you do Chocolate; turn up the Bottom of a clean Hair-ſieve, and as the Froth riſes on your Cream take it off with a Spoon and lay it on your Sieve, and when it will caſt no more Froth, pour it into the Diſh, and heap it up with the Froth.

To make Currant Cream.

TAKE a Quart of Cream and put into a China-bowl, and mill it up in the above Manner, laying the Froth on the Bottom of a Hair-ſieve; and when you have Froth ſufficient to make a large Heap, take a Quarter of a Pound of Currant-gelly and mix with the Cream; put it into the Diſh, and heap it up with the Froth.

Lemon Cream.

TAKE a Quart of Cream and ſweeten to your Taſte, ſqueeze into it the Juice of a Lemon, and put it into a China or Delf-bowl, and mull as aforeſaid, putting the Froth upon it; cut the Lemon

mon into ſmall Shreds, and lay the Froth over and round the Diſh.

A Whip Poſſet.

TAKE a Quart of Cream and ſweeten to your Taſte, add a Glaſs of Orange-flower Water to it; then put a Pint of Sack into a Quart Glaſs-bowl, and mill up the Cream, lay the Froth on a Hair-ſieve to drain the Milk from it, and let it lie on it Half an Hour before you lay it on the Sack; be careful to keep a ſteady Hand as you drop it from the Spoon, and heap the Glaſs-bowl with Froth.

A Crow Crant.

TAKE wet or dry Sweet-meats, aud fill a Diſh as full as for a Pye; then take a deep Diſh of the ſame Breadth of the other that your Sweet-meats are in, turn it upſide down, and cover it with a Sheet of Paſte of Milk and Sugar boil'd, wrought with Flour; then roll it out thin, and cut it out in various Shapes and Forms, bake it on the Diſh, and take great Care not to have any burnt Spots on it; when it is enough take it out of the Diſh, and ſet it upon the Sweet-meats.

Sweet-meat Tarts.

TURN up the Bottom of a Tart-pan, and cut out of a Sheet of common raiſed Paſte with your Jager-irons into Strings, no broader than Tape three Yards a Penny, rub the Outſide of your Tart-pan with a little Butter, and lay over your Paſte, croſs it into Diamond Figures, and bake it in as many as will make a Diſh; put preſerv'd Plumbs, Cherries, or Gooſeberries into Saucers, and ſet the Diamond-paſte Covers over your Preſerves.

To

To make Glazed Tarts.

FILL your Tart-pans with Sweet-meats, make a Paſte of double-refin'd Sugar beat and ſifted, take the Whites of three Eggs and a little Orange-flower Water, and beat an Hour to an Icing; then lay round the Edge of your Tart-pan a little of this Icing, and cover it with Wafer-paper, and with a Pair of Sciſſors clip the Wafer-paper cloſe to the Edge of the Tart-pan; then lay over a thin Icing and ſet it in a ſlow Oven five Minutes: Do as many as your Icing will make. You are not to put any Syrup in with your preſerv'd Plumbs, Gooſeberries, or Cherries, or any other Thing.

To make Tart Puff-paſte.

MIX Flour and fair Water into Paſte, take the ſame Weight of Butter and divide it into three Parts, roll out the Paſte three Times, and lay on one Part of the Butter each Time, daſhing on a little Flour over the Butter every Time: This Paſte is for fine Puddings and Tarts, but is too rich for Pyes.

Criſp Paſte for Tarts.

TAKE three Pints of Flour, and five Ounces of Butter, rub the Butter into the Flour as ſmall as poſſible, ſo that the leaſt Piece of Butter cannot be ſeen, ſo that all the Flour be as if no Butter was in it by being ſo mealy; then take ſix Eggs, leaving out the Whites of Two, and put three Spoonfuls of Water, mix this Paſte, and roll it out almoſt as as thin as Wafers; bake it criſp, and if it be kept till it ſoftens, ſetting it a while before the Fire criſpens it again.

To

To make Light Wigs.

RUB ſix Ounces of Butter into three Pounds of
fine Flour, and take a Quart of Milk, beat up
three Eggs, and half a Pound of Powder-ſugar;
warm the Milk and mix with the Sugar, Flour, and
Eggs well together; add two Spoonfuls of freſh
Yeſt, mix all well together, and ſet it an Hour before the Fire to riſe; then put half an Ounce of
Carroway-ſeeds, and roll out your Wigs; let them
ſtand on a Board before the Fire to riſe, before you
ſet them into the Oven.

Bath Cakes.

TAKE a Pound of Flour and a Pint of Milk,
beat up three Eggs with a Spoonful of Yeſt,
mix all together and ſet in a Bowl before the Fire;
when it is riſen very high, take half a Pound of
Butter and half a Pound of Sugar, and work into
it with your Hands; add a little Roſe-water, grate
a Nutmeg, beat a little Cinnamon and mix thereto;
then bake them in Queen-cake Pans, ſome plain,
and ſome you may put Currants into.

A Pound Cake.

TAKE a Pound of Loaf-ſugar beat and ſift it
through a Sieve, add to it a Pound of Eggs
and a little Roſe-water, beat it till it turns very thick
and white; then take a Pound of Butter and beat
up with your Hand to a Cream, the Eggs and Sugar beat with a Whisk; then take a Pound of very
fine Flour, dry it before the Fire, and mix all with
your Hand half an Hour; add to it an Ounce of
Carroway-ſeeds, put it into a Pan and bake it an
Hour and a Half.

A

A Fruit Cake.

TAKE eight Pounds of Currants and pick them clean, ſtone three Pounds of Raiſins and cut them ſmall, beat Cinnamon, Mace, and Nutmeg of each half an Ounce, Cloves a Quarter of an Ounce, a Pound and a Half of *Jourdon* Almonds blanched and cut very ſmall, and the hot Spice to be powdered; then take three Pounds of Butter and beat to Cream, mix it with fourteen Eggs, and take four Pounds of Flour and mix with the Butter and Eggs; add a Jill of Brandy, a Jill of Sack, and a little new Yeſt, beat it till it is light; then put in the hot Spices and cut Almonds, mix them well together, and then put in the Fruit, beat and mix all well together; then cut a Pound of Orange and Lemon-peal, half a Pound of Citron cut into thin Slices, and greaſe your Pan with Butter; lay in your Cake at three Lairs, on each lay the Lemon and Orange-peal, and Citron intermix'd; when it is all in and your Cake pack'd cloſe in the Cake-pan, ſet it into an Oven: It will take four Hours baking.

To make Queen Cakes.

TAKE half a Pound of Butter and beat up to Cream, beat and ſift half a Pound of Loaf-ſugar, beat four Eggs and mix with the Sugar, and beat the Eggs and Sugar a Quarter of an Hour before you mix your Butter; then weigh half a Pound of Flour, ſetting it before the Fire on a Diſh ten Minutes before you mix your Butter, and ſo mix all together; add to it a Glaſs of Orange-flower Water, and beat it half an Hour longer with your Hand; then put them into Pans and bake them in a ſlow Oven, which is much better for theſe Cakes than any other.

T

To preſerve Plumbs.

TAKE large Magnum Plumbs and let their Stalks be kept on, and to every Pound of Plumbs take a Pound and a half of double-refined Sugar; then to every Pound of Sugar put a Jill of Water, and put it into a clean Preſerving-pan, boil it near to candy Height, and with a Penknife make a very little Slit at the End of each Plumb and take off the Skin, ſet them upon their Ends with the Stalk-end uppermoſt in an Earthen-pot, and pour on your Syrup to the Plumbs, cover them up and let them ſtand three Days, by which Time the Syrup will be thin, you muſt put it into your Pan and boil it up till it will rope, pour it upon the Plumbs and let them ſtand a Week; if your Syrup be thin, boil it up again to a ropy Thickneſs, and pour upon your Plumbs, and let them ſtand a Fortnight; if the Syrup keeps Subſtance, put up your Plumbs in Pots, cover them with Papers and Bladders, and keep them for your Uſe.

To candy the above. Plumbs.

TAKE Magnum Plumbs, cut off all the Plumb, but leave the Stone and Stalk together; the Plumbs muſt not be ripe, but at their full Growth; take great Care to have a ſharp Knife, and not to ſeparate the Stone from the Stalk; take the Weight of the Plumbs of double-refined Sugar, put the Plumbs and Sugar into a Pot, and ſet them into a ſlow Oven two Hours; ſet the Plumb-ſtones and Stalks into the Sun to dry; then take out the Plumbs and mix them with their Syrup, put them through a Hair-ſieve and preſs through all their Pulp, and put into your Preſerving-pan, and boil it to a Plumb-paſte; make on the Stalk the Form of

a

a Plumb with this Paſte, and dry them in cool O-
vens or in the Sun; when they are thoroughly dried
boil up double-refined Sugar, candy Height, and dip
in each Plumb one by one, ſet them on their Ends
on a flat-bottomed Delft-diſh, and when the Candy
is dry, take up each Plumbs with a thin ſharp Knife.

To *preſerve green* Gages.

TAKE to every Pound of green Gages a Pound
and a half of Sugar; take the Plumbs and ſet
on a ſlow Fire to ſcald, when they are ready take
off all their Skins, and put the Plumbs into the Water they were ſcalded in; add to them a little Piece
of Allum beat to a Powder, cover the Plumbs with
Plumb Tree-leaves, and ſet them a great Diſtance
from the Fire till they be green; then take them
out, ſet them on a flat-bottomed Diſh with their
Stalks up, and when they are drained put them into a broad Pot in the ſame Way; boil up your Sugar to a thick Syrup, pour it over your Plumbs,
cover them up, and let them ſtand two Days; boil
up the Syrup again till it will rope, pour it on your
Plumbs, and let them ſtand a Week; boil the Syrup as ſtrong up as before, pour it over the Plumbs;
when they have ſtood a Fortnight, if the Syrup
be any thinner boil it up again; then you may put
them into Pots for Uſe, and tie them cloſe with
White-paper and Bladders.

Currant Gelly.

STRIP the Currants of their Stalks, when they
are thoroughly ripe, put them into a Jarr, and
ſet them into an Oven or a Pot of hot Water; when
the Berries are thoroughly hot, ſo as to diſcharge their
Juice, ſtrain it through a Flannel-bag, and to every
Jill of this Juice put a Pound of double-refined Sugar;

put

put it into a Brass-pan clean scoured, and boil it over a Stove till it becomes a thick Gelly, scumming it all the Time; then put it in Glasses or Pots for Use. If you have any Rasps you may put a Quart into the Currants; the Currants after the Juice is run from them, will make a small Wine.

To make Rasp Jam.

AFTER you have picked all the Worms and Greens out of the Rasps, take their Weight of Loaf-sugar, and put into a Preserving-pan; set it over a clear Stove, let it boil till you see it stiff, and take great Care to keep stirring it; when it begins to fly in Sparks, take it off, and put it in Pots or Glasses; cover it with White-paper dipp'd in Brandy, and put Bladders over it.

To preserve Rasps *whole.*

TAKE a Pint of the Juice of Currants; add to it three Pound of double-refined Sugar, put into a Preserving-pan upon a clear Stove, and boil it to a very strong Gelly; then have a Quart of fine pick'd Rasps, put them into the Gelly, let them boil five Minutes, and put them into Glasses.

To preserve Gooseberries.

TAKE Gooseberries when at their full Growth, cut a Nick on each Side, and with a Pin pick out the Seeds; to every Pound of Berries, take a Pound and a Half of double-refined Sugar; put a Jill of Water to every Pound, and boil your Sugar to a thick Syrup; put your Gooseberries into a Pot, pour upon them this Syrup, and let them stand two Days; if the Syrup be thin, boil it up again till it be ropy, and then pour it on them,
and

and let them stand a Week; then boil it up, and put in the Berries, let them boil three Minutes; put them into your Glasses, and keep them for Use.

To *preserve* Currants *in* Strops.

TAKE red Currants, and with a Pin make a Hole at the End of each Currant, pick out all the Seeds, and make a Syrup of double-refin'd Sugar and pour upon the Berries, and let it stand two Days; then strip as many Currants as will make a Jill of Juice, pour the Syrup from the Berries in Strops, and boil up with this Currant-juice, till it becomes a weak Gelly; then take it off the Fire, put in your Currants in Strops, and put them into Glasses, and keep them for Use.

To *preserve* Peaches.

TAKE green Peaches when a Pin will run through the Stone, put them into a Pan with Water, set them on a flow Fire, and let them stand till they are scalding hot; when they are so done, take them out of the Water, take off the Skins, and put them into the Water you took them out of, cover them with Peach-leaves, put a little Allum into the Pan, and cover it very close; set it on a very flow Fire, and let it stand till the Peaches are green; then take them out of the Water, to every Pound of Peaches take a Pound and a half of double-refined Sugar; add Water to the Sugar, and boil in a clear Brass-pan till it is a rich Syrup; put your Peaches into a Pot, pour this Syrup upon them, cover them close, and let them stand a Week; take the Syrup into the Pan again, and boil it till it will rope; then put in your Peaches and give them a boil, not exceeding three Minutes; then put the Peaches into Pots, covering them with Syrup,

and

and paper them up; if the Syrup turns thin, boil it
up till it is rich, and pour upon them again: Keep
them for Deferts, Sweet-meat Tarts, or fend them
up in Sweet-meat Glaffes. You do Apricots, and
Nectars in the fame Manner.

To make Goofeberry Wine.

TAKE Cryftal Goofeberries, pick and bruife
them in a Wooden-bowl or Mortar, and to e-
very Gallon of bruifed Berries put two Quarts of
Water, and let them ftand in a clean Tub twenty-
four Hours; then ftrain them through a Hair-fieve,
take out the Skins and Seeds, but be fure to prefs
through all the Pulp you poffibly can; to every
Gallon of Liquor add four Pounds of double-refined
Sugar; tun it up into a Brandy-cask if you have
one of the Size, and bung it down, but leave the
Spile-hole open; when it has done fomenting, put
in the Spile, and let it ftand fix Months; then bottle it.

To make red Currant Wine.

GATHER your Currants when they are full
ripe, pick off their Stalks, and bruize them
with a Wooden-peftle; to every Gallon of bruifed
Berries put a Gallon of Spring-water, and let it ftand
two Days, ftirring it every fix Hours; then ftrain
it through a Hair-fieve, take out the Skins and
Seeds, and prefs the Pulp through the Sieve; to e-
very Gallon of Liquor put in three Pound and a
half of double-refined Sugar, and to every twenty
Quarts add a Pint of the beft *French* Brandy; then
tun it and bung it down, leaving open your Spile-
hole; when it has done fomenting clofe it up, and
in four Months you may bottle it off. Black Currants are done after the fame Manner.

To

To make Cowſlip Wine.

PICK your Cowſlips, to every Pound of Flowers take a Gallon of Water, and beat the Flowers in a Marble Mortar; then mix them with the Water, to every ſix Gallons of Water add a Dozen of *Seville* Oranges, ſqueeze in their Juice, let ſix of their Skins be put in with the Juice, and let it ſtand all Night in the Tub, then ſtrain them through a Sieve; to every Gallon of Liquor add four Pounds of double-refined Sugar, and ſtir all well together; add two Spoonfuls of Gile-yeaſt, and let it ſtand all Night in the Tub; tun it up into a Cask, adding a Pint of Brandy to every ſix Gallons of Wine, bung it down cloſe, leaving the Spile-hole open till it be done working; then cloſe it up, and in ſix Months Time you may bottle it.

To make Baum Wine.

TAKE Baum at full Growth, the firſt Cutting, and beat in a Mortar or Wooden-bowl; to every Pound of Baum put a Gallon of Water, and let the Water and Baum ſtand twenty-four Hours; then ſtrain it through a Flannel-bag, and ſqueeze its Juice out of it; to every Gallon of Liquor add three Pounds of double-refined Sugar, and ſtir it till all the Sugar is mix'd well with the Liquor; then add to it a Jill of Ale-yeaſt, very freſh off the Fats, and tun it up, leaving the Spile-hole open, till it be done fomenting; then cloſe it up, and it will be ready in four Months for bottling.

To make Raiſin Wine.

TAKE *Malaga* Raiſins, and to every Stone of Raiſins put ſix Quarts of Water in an open headed Cask, and let them ſtand twelve Days, ſtir-
ing

ing them every Day; then ſtrain the Raiſins all out
of the Tub, ſqueeze them well in your Hands as
you take them out, and then take a clean Hair-
cloth, put as many Raiſins into it as will preſs without letting any of the Skins out, and the Pulp thereof put into your Liquor; after you have ſtrain'd it
through a Hair-ſieve, tun it up, and bung it, leave
out the Spile-pin till it has done fomenting, and in
ſix Months Time it will be fit for Uſe; but if not
fine in that Time, if you have half a Hogſhead of
Wine, take an Ounce of Iſing-glaſs, cut it with a
Knife, and put it into a Quart of rough Cider; cut
the ſmall End off a Whiſk, and beat this up every
Day with the Whiſk, till all the Glaſs is diſſolved,
it will be all thick as Calf's Feet Gelly is when it
is cold; then ſtrain it through a fine Wood-ſieve,
draw out a little of the Wine and mix with it, and
as much more of the Wine as the Cider and Iſing-
glaſs; then pour in the Iſing-glaſs and Wine, ſtir-
ing it with a Stick not above a Quarter of a Yard
within the Cask, and round the Cask; then bung
it cloſe down, and it will be fine in forty-eight
Hours: This Method will fine any of the above
Wines.

To make Orange Wine.

TO ſix Gallons of Water take three Dozen of
Oranges, and ſqueeze out their Juice; take the
Rind of twelve Oranges and put into the Water
with the Juice, and let it ſtand two Days, ſtirring
it every ſix Hours; then ſtrain it through a Hair-
ſieve, and preſs the Juice of the Oranges all through
the Sieve; to every Gallon of Liquor add four
Pound of Loaf-ſugar, and put two Spoonfuls of
Yeaſt freſh off the Gile-fat to it; tun it up, put a
Quart of Brandy thereto, leave the Spile-hole open
till it be done working, and it will be fit for bottling in four Months.

To make Cherry Wine.

TAKE twenty Pounds of *Morella* Cherries full ripe, a d bruiſe them; take two Gallons of red Currants ſtripp'd from the Stalks, and bruiſed with a Wooden-peſtle, and put them in a clean Veſſel open headed; to every Gallon add a Gallon of boiling Water, ſtir all together, and let it ſtand forty-eight Hours, ſtirring it up every ſix Hours; then ſtrain it through a Hair-ſieve, and to every Gallon of Liquor add three Pounds of double-refined Sugar; put it into a Brandy-cask, leave the Spile-pin open till it be done working, and in three Months you may bottle it off.

To make Elder Wine.

STRIP your Elder-berries off the Stalks, put them into a large deep Earthen-pot, cover it cloſe, and ſet it in an Oven all Night; then take it out of the Oven, and ſtrain off the Juice into a clean Pot; to every Gallon of Juice put a Gallon of Water, and to every Gallon of Liquor put three Pounds of Loaf-ſugar; put it into a Cask that has had Brandy in it, bung it down, leaving the Spile-hole open, and when it has done fomenting, cloſe it up.

To make Bramble Wine.

INFUSE your Bramble-berries as above directed; to every Gallon of Juice add two Gallons of Water, and to every Gallon of Liquor put three Pounds of Loaf-ſugar; ſtir it well till all the Sugar is diſſolved, and let it ſtand twenty Hours in the Tub you mix it in; then tun it up into a Cask, leaving your Spile-hole open, and when it has done fomenting cloſe it up; it will be ready for bottling in ſix Months, and fit for drinking.

To

To pickle Muſhrooms.

TAKE the cloſe Buttons, cut off their Stalks, and put them into Water an Hour; then take a Bruſh made of Rice, ſtrain and waſh your Muſhrooms with this Bruſh, and put as much Water as the Muſhrooms require to cover them, ſo that this Bruſh takes the Scurf off the Muſhrooms; then give them plenty of clean Water, and waſh them with the Bruſh as before; then take them into a clean Cullender, having a clean Pan that juſt holds the Muſhrooms, put them into it, and cover it cloſe; ſet it on a clear Fire with nothing but the Muſhrooms, which will diſcharge as much of their own Liquor as will cover them, and let them boil in this Liquor five Minutes; in which Time make a Brine of Salt and Water ſo ſtrong as to bear an Egg; then drain the Liquor from the Muſhrooms, put them into this Salt-brine, and let them ſtand five Days, ſtirring them every Day; make another Brine as ſtrong as the former, put in the Muſhrooms, let them ſtand a Week longer, and this is phyſicking the Muſhrooms; then add to them ſome diſtilled Vinegar, and let them lie fourteen Days, after all bottle them; every Bottle will take a Jill of diſtilled Vinegar, and put two Blades of Mace into each Bottle: This will keep either cloſe or open in Bottles or Jarrs; now the Juice that the Muſhrooms diſcharges in the Pan, is the beſt of Catchup; if you have a Pint of it, add three Spoonfuls of Beef-brine, if it be freſh and perfectly ſweet, alſo Mace, Nutmeg, Cloves, and Pepper powdered, and boil it, filtering it through a Flannel-bag: This will be proper for White-ſauces.

To

To *pickle* Walnuts.

TAKE Walnuts when they are almoſt at their
full Growth, but that a Pin will run through
them; then pick off their Stalks, rub them with a
coarſe Cloth, make a Brine of Salt, and let it be ſo
ſtrong as to bear an Egg; then put in your Walnuts and lay a Board upon them to keep them under the Brine, and let them lie in this Brine ſix
Days; then make a freſh Brine, pour off this from
them and put in the freſh Brine, let them ſtand ten
Days longer, and then take and dry them with a
coarſe Cloth: To every Hundred of Walnuts take
a Jill of Muſtard-ſeed, lay your Walnuts in Lairs,
and upon every Lair ſtrew your Muſtard proporti-
onably, and when your Jarr is full have ſome of the
beſt Beer-vinegar and put in; for every Hundred of
Walnuts have *Jamaica* and Black-pepper of each
an Ounce, Mace and Nutmeg of each half an Ounce,
and boil up in the Vinegar, pour it boiling upon
the Walnuts, and put a Bladder over them; don't
uſe them till the Bitter be overcome by the Pickle
and hot Spices: This Pickle makes Sauces richer
than Catchup made of Muſhrooms.

To *make* Walnut Catchup.

TAKE four Hundred of Walnuts, ſuch as before deſcribed, and with a ſharp Penknife cut
off all the pulpy Part till you are at the inner Shell,
and be careful to keep that whole, beat the green
Pulp in a Mortar, and to every Pint of the Pulp
add a Spoonful of freſh Beef-brine, and let it lie
20 Hours; then take the Shells that you cut the
green Part of the Walnut from, and put them into

a

a Jarr, make a Brine of Milk-whey, pour it boiling
hot upon the Shells, and let them ſtand twenty-four
Hours; then take your Walnut-pulp and ſtrain it
through a clean coarſe Linen-cloth, ſqueeze all the
Juice you can poſſibly get out of it, and to every
Pint of this Juice add Nutmeg, Mace, and Black-
pepper of each a Quarter of an Ounce, and half
that Quantity of Cloves; then boil it up, but do not
make any uſe of it till the Bitter is gone off: A
Tea-ſpoonful of this will make Sauce rich for Fiſh
or any Made-diſh, nor is there any Thing ſo agreeable to the Taſte, for I never knew that the moſt
delicate Palate objected it, nor the tendereſt Stomach
was offended therewith: Then you take the Walnuts out of the Whey, and with a Flannel-rag waſh
all the Scurf off them into clear Water; then put
them into Bottles wi h wide Mouths, fill them up
with diſtill'd Vinegar that has been diſtill'd from
Beer-vinegar, and hot Spices: This is a delicious
pretty Pickle that very few are acquainted with.

To pickle Onions.

TAKE Onions no larger than ſmall Nutmegs,
pour boiling Water upon them, and take off
their brown Coat; put the Onions into a Brine of
Milk, with Salt and Water into a Pan, and take the
Onions out of the Milk-brine into a Cullender;
when the Salt and Water boils put them in, and let
them boil two Minutes; then take them out of the
Water and lay them on a Cloth to cool; put them
into Bottles with diſtill'd Vinegar, and keep them
for Uſe.

To pickle Colliflowers.

LET your Colliflowers be very white and without Frickles, and let them be cloſe; cut them
into Buds and boil them in a Brine of Salt and
Water

Water one Minute; then take them out and lay them to cool, when they are cold put them into Jarrs, and fill them with diſtill'd Vinegar; then tye them down cloſe with a Bladder and Pack-thread for Uſe.

To pickle Turnips.

CUT your Turnips into various Shapes, that you may have them for Garniſhing, and cut them a Quarter of an Inch thick; let your Turnips be clear of Worm-eaten, and let them boil a Minute in Salt and Water; then take them out into a coarſe Cloth, and when they are cold and all the Water drain'd out put them into a Glaſs-jarr, fill them up with diſtilled Vinegar; cover them cloſe with a Bladder, and keep them for Uſe.

To pickle Kidney Beans.

TAKE Whey after it is ſcalded and the Curds from it, make a Brine ſo ſtrong as to bear an Egg, let your Beans be young and dry pull'd, put them into the Whey-brine till their Colour is diſcharg'd; when they are of a bright Yellow, take them out of the Whey into a Cullender, and dry them with a coarſe Cloth; then put them into a Braſs-pan and cover them with Beer-vinegar, put in ſome Dill, and cover them cloſe down, put Paper round the Edge of your Cover, and ſet the Pan a good Diſtance from the Fire, if it be hot; but if ſlow, it need not be at ſo great a Diſtance, and let it ſtand till the Beans turn graſs Green; then take them out of this Vinegar and put them into a Jarr, and make Pickle of freſh Beer-vinegar, *Jamaica* and Black-pepper, and Race-ginger boil'd up, pour it upon your Beans, and keep them for Uſe. The aforeſaid Receipts is a Rule to pickle Girkins, Cucumbers, Parſley, Reddiſh-pods, Aſtertion-buds, Broom-

Broom-buds, or Burtree-buds: So there is no need
of telling the Tale oftner over than is neceſſary.

To *mango* Cucumbers.

TAKE large Cucumbers and cut a long narrow
Piece out of each, with the Mouth of a Tea-
ſpoon pick out all the Seeds and Pulp of it, gather
out all the Seeds and mix them with white Muſtard-
ſeed, Aſtertion-buds, Shalot, and ſome Salt ; fill the
Cucumbers with this Mixture and put them cloſe
down in a Jarr, boil up Beer-vinegar, Salt, *Jamaica*
and Black-pepper, with Race-ginger, and pour upon
the Mangoes, cover them cloſe and let them ſtand
two Days ; then boil up the Pickle again, and repeat
it till your Mangoes are green, and keep them for Uſe.

To *mango* Apples.

THERE is a long green Apple call'd a Finger,
take of this Sort, and with a Penknife cut a
round Piece out at each End, with an Apple-ſcope
take out all the Core, and fill the Place with Horſe-
radiſh, White-muſtard, and a little Mace ; put the
Pieces on at each End from whence they were taken,
and ſew it up with a Needle and Thread, pack them
cloſe up into a Jarr, and boil Beer-vinegar with *Jamaica* and Black-pepper, Race-ginger and Salt, and
pour it boiling hot upon the Mangoes ; let them
ſtand, and repeat the boiling of the Vinegar till you
ſee your Mangoes turn green ; then cover them with
a Bladder, and keep them for Uſe.

To *mango* Millons.

TAKE little Millons of the latter Growth, when
the firſt Growth is over, and cut a long Piece
out of the Side ; take out the Seed, and put your
Millons

Millons in Whey till they have diſcharg'd their Colour; then take as much Vinegar as you have to
Cucumbers to green them, and cover the Millons
with it, place them at a little Diſtance from the
Fire till they are green; then take them up, and
when they are cold, take the Seeds you took out of
them, and mix with white Muſtard, Horſe-radiſh
cut ſmall, and Afterſion-ſeed; mix all well, fill up
your Millons, and put the Pieces you cut out into
their proper Places; take four Yards a Penny Tape
to roll up the Millons, and put them into a Jarr;
boil up Beer-vinegar, *Jamaica* and Black-pepper,
and Race-ginger, and pour boiling upon the Millons; cover them with a Paper, and keep them cloſe
for Uſe.

To pickle Dutch Cabbage.

TAKE a red Cabbage, cut it into four Quarters,
take out the Core, with a ſharp Knife cut
your Cabbage, lay it into a Wooden-diſh, mix it
with Salt, and let it lie five Days, turning it with
your Hands every Day; when it has lain the above
Time, take up a Handful and ſqueeze with all your
Strength, and when one Handful is done take another, till you have ſqueezed it all; then ſet upon a
clear Fire a broad Pan, and boil as much Beer-vinegar as will cover the Cabbage, and have *Jamaica*
and Black-pepper, and Race-ginger; when it boils
put in the Cabbage, and let it not boil above a Minute; then take it up, put it into a Jarr, and keep
it cloſe covered for Uſe: You may put into it ſome
red Beat Root.

To pickle Pumpkins.

TAKE a Pumpkin and cut into half Inch Slices,
after you have taken out all the Seed, cut it into various Forms, ſo as to make ornamental for garniſhing

nifhing fuch as carved Work, &c. the Outfide is a
bright rich yellow; boil White-wine Vinegar and
hot Spices, and pour upon your Mango into a Jarr
three fundry Times, and keep for Ufe.

To pickle Barberry-berries.

TAKE Barberry-berries when they are full ripe,
pick all the Leaves from off the Stalks, take
all the fmall Barberry-berries and beat in a Mortar;
then make a Brine of Salt fo ftrong as to bear an
Egg, and boil the beaten Barberry-berries in it, put
them through a Flannel-bag, and boil it up again;
powder Two-pennyworth of Cocheneal and put to
it; then put the Berries into a Jarr, and pour this
Brine boiling upon them, and lay a Piece of Flannel
over the Barberry-berries within the Jarr; cover the
Jarr, and keep them for garnifhing Fifh, Fowl, Rabbets, or any other Made-difh.

To make Mackroons.

TAKE a Pound of *Jourdon* Almonds, blanch and
beat them in a Marble Mortar to a Pafte, take
the Whites of five Eggs, and a Pound of beat and
fifted Loaf-fugar, and mix with the Whites of the
Eggs; beat the Sugar and Whites one Quarter of
an Hour with a Whisk, before you mix it with the
Almond-pafte; then add to it a Glafs of Orange-
flower Water, and beat all well with a Wooden-
peftle a Quarter of an Hour; lay fome Wafer-paper
upon Wires, and drop the Mackroons on the Paper:
Set them in a fharp Oven, and a Quarter of an
Hour will bake them.

To make Ratafia Drops.

TAKE a Pound of *Jourdon* Almonds and half a
Pound of bitter Almonds, blanch and beat them
to Paſte; take a Pound and a half of beaten and
ſifted fine Loaf-ſugar, add three Eggs and beat the
Eggs, Sugar and Almond-paſte all well together till
they become a very ſtiff Paſte, add to it a Glaſs of
Ratafia or *French* Brandy: You muſt have a Marble
Mortar for your Purpoſe, and obſerve to have your
Ingredients not only work'd to a proper Stiffneſs,
but alſo to a very fine Smoothneſs; then drop it on
Cap-paper in Drops as big as large Nutmegs, bake
them brown in a ſharp Oven, and keep them for
Uſe.

To make a Biſcuit Cake.

BEAT and ſift a Pound of Loaf-ſugar, take a
Pound of Eggs and beat with the Sugar till it
is thick, add to it a Pound of fine *London* Flour;
put it into a Cake-pan, after you have rubb'd the Pan
with Butter, and bake it in a ſlow Oven.

To make Biſcuit Drops.

TAKE a Pound of Loaf-ſugar well beat and
ſifted through a Hair-ſieve, beat four Eggs
with the Sugar till it is very white and thick; take
a Pound and a Quarter of the fineſt *London* Flour,
and let it ſtand drying before the Fire a Quarter of
an Hour; then mix it with the Eggs and Sugar,
adding a Glaſs of Orange-flour Water to it, and
when it is well mix'd drop it on Gray-paper, and
bake them in a ſlow Oven: Be exceeding careful to
take your Papers off whilſt hot, for if they are ſuffer-
ed to cool, they will by no Means part with their
Paper.

A P-

APPENDIX.

Pigeons *paradised.*

PICK, singe, and wash six Pigeons, cut up their Backs and take out the Bones; then cut the Livers small with a Quarter of a Pound of Beef-suet, pounding them well in a Mortar, steep the Crumb of a Halfpenny Roll in Cream and beat with it; add to it the Yolks of four Eggs boiled hard; and season it with Mace, Nutmeg, Pepper, and Salt; add green Thyme, Sweet-marjoram, and Parsley; break two Eggs and mix it well together; then divide it equally amongst the Pigeons, after you have dried them well with a clean coarse Cloth; put the Stuffing equally within them, and put them in the Form they were before you boned them; lay them in a flat-bottomed Earthen-dish, and rub the Breast of each Pigeon with Butter, throwing over all some grated Bread and green Parsley; then rub some Butter on white Paper and lay over them, and set them an Hour in an Oven; then take a Quarter of a Pound of Rice, boil, and drain it dry in a Hair-sieve; colour one Half of it Green with the Juice of Sorrel, and the other Half let be White, and lay it round the Dish-rim in various Forms; and have half a Hundred Asparagus boiled, and cut the green Tops, and stew in good Gravy thickned with Butter and Flour, pour it on the Dish; lay on the Pigeons with Sippets and green Parsley, and serve it up.

Pigeons

Pigeons *in Blankets.*

PICK and waſh your Pigeons clean, and dry
them: For three Pigeons, take the Yolks of
ſix hard boiled Eggs cut ſmall, add green Thyme,
Sweet-marjoram, and Parſley ſhred fine, and take the
Bulk of a Hen's Egg of Butter, and work up all the
Ingredients, which divide equally amongſt and put
into the Pigeons; then roll out three Sheets of cold
Paſte, into each Sheet roll a Pigeon, and tie it tight
in a Cloth: Boil them an Hour and a Half; then
take off the Cloths, and lay them in a Diſh. For
Sauce, Gravy and Butter.

A ſavoury Pigeon Pye.

MAKE a raiſed Cruſt, that is, a ſtanding Cruſt;
for four Pigeons, make three Corners and
one in the Middle, and when it is cold, take ſome
ſavoury Force-meat and draw all over the Inſide;
bone the Pigeons, and rub them on the Inſide with
Yolk of Egg, and lay on ſome of the Force-meat;
put them as for baking, and let their Breaſt be uppermoſt; then put on the Lid, and let them ſtand
two Hours in a moderate Oven: Then have a Jill
of Gravy and Butter, and pour into it.

Another Pigeon Pye.

TAKE ſix Pigeons, pick and waſh them clean,
cut off their Feet and Pinions; take half a
Pound of Butter, and work up in it as much Pepper
and Salt as you think reaſonable to ſeaſon them;
then make a Sheet of cold Paſte, and lay a Rim
round the Edge of the Diſh, and lay in your Pigeons,
after you have put an equal Quantity of Butter and
Seaſoning within each, put the Gizzards, Livers,
and Pinions into the Diſh, add a Pint of Water, and
lay a Sheet of Paſte over all: Bake it an Hour and
a Half in a moderate Oven; when it is drawn, put
half a Jill of good Gravy into it.

A

A white *Fricassey* of Eggs.

BOIL six Eggs hard, and take out their Yolks, cut the Whites very small; take a clean Frying-pan and heat some Butter hot, but take Care not to brown it; then drop in six Eggs and fry them White, lay them on a clean Tin-pan and set them before the Fire; rub your Frying-pan clean, and put more Butter into it, and fry as many more Eggs in the above Manner, and lay them into the same Pan, then take a Knife and cut off all the Rags; when you have trimmed them, take half a Wine-pint of sweet Cream and a Quarter of a Pound sweet Butter, wrought in Flour; put your fried Eggs into a Hash-pan, add to them the Cream and Butter, with a little powdered Mace, grated Nutmeg, and Salt; then toss it up, and when it boils take it off the Fire, and squeeze in the Juice of a Lemon; toss it up, and lay the Whites round the Dish; cut some Parsley, then pour in the Fricassey; lay the hard Yolks over it, and serve it up.

A brown *Fricassey* of Eggs.

TAKE six Eggs, break and separate the Yolks from the Whites; tie the Yolks in a Linen-rag and boil them hard, cut them small, and grate the Crumb of a Halfpenny Roll, and mix with the shred Yolks; add Nutmeg, Pepper, Salt, Thyme, and Sweet-marjoram cut small, and rub the Bulk of a Nutmeg of Butter into the Mixture; take a raw Egg and work it up, dusting a little Flour over it, roll it into small Balls, and rub a Plate with Butter, then set them to brown before the Fire or in an Oven: Beat the Whites with a Spoonful of Cream, add Nutmeg, Salt, and Parsley cut very small; then take a very small Bladder and pour in the Whites, leaving a little for them to rise in boiling; then take a thick Slice of sweet Butter in a Frying-pan over a

sharp

ſharp Stove or clear Fire, brown the Butter, and drop ſix Eggs, fry them brown on both Sides; then pour out the Eggs and Butter into a clean Haſh-pan, and fry ſix more Eggs in the above Manner, and put them to the other Eggs; then half a Jill of Wa-ter, of Walnut Pickle, Catchup, and Muſhrooms, each a Spoonful. Thicken it with Butter and Flour.

A Pallateen *of* Eggs.

BEAT tweive Eggs, and take out the Crumb of a Penny Loaf, add to it a Jill of Rheniſh Wine, and mix it well with the Eggs; boil ſix Artichokes, take the Buttoms and cut ſmall, and mix with the Eggs; ſeaſon them with Mace, Nutmeg, and Salt, and mix them all well together: Greaſe a round Ba-ſon that will juſt hold them, and pour them into it, lay three thin Slices of Butter over all, and ſet it an Hour in a ſlow Oven; then take half a Hundred freſh Oyſters and waſh them clean in Water, lay them on a clean Board, and ſeaſon them with Black-pepper and Salt, and drudge ſome Flour over them; then take a Quarter of a Pound of Butter in a clean Fry-ing-pan over a clear Stove or brisk Fire, let the But-ter be brown when you put in the Oyſters, and turn them; then add to them half a Jill of Water, a Spoonful of Catchup, and thicken it with Flour and Butter; then turn the Eggs out of the Baſon on the Middle of the Diſh, pour over it the Ragoo: Gar-niſh with Barberry-berries and Parſley, and ſend it up.

Eggs *a la Mode.*

TAKE ten Eggs and beat them well, ſoak the Crumb of a Penny Loaf in Cream and beat with them, boil a Hundred of Aſparagus, cut the green Ends ſmall, and mix with the above, add Nutmeg, Pepper and Salt; when you have mixt them well, butter a Tin-pan, and lay a thin Sheet of Puff-paſte in it, pour on your Eggs, and throw

over

over ſome grated Bread and melted Butter, ſet it in
an Oven; then take a Quart of Water, ſlice a Carrot, and put to it a Faggot of ſweet Herbs, Horſe-
radiſh and Shalots, let it boil to half a Pint; then
ſtrain it in a clean Pan, add to it two Spoonfuls of
Catchup; and take a Slice of Butter in a Frying-
pan, brown it over a clear Fire, toſs up the Sauce
in the Frying-pan, and ſo put it in the Sauce-pan;
thicken it with Butter and Flour, and have ſome
Force-meat Balls as before directed; then take out
your Eggs and cut them into Dices, leaving a large
One for the Middle; then diſh it up, pour over the
Sauce, ſtrew over the Force-meat Balls, and ſome
pickled Muſhrooms. Garniſh with green Parſley.

Another Way to a la Mode Eggs.

BREAK ſixteen Eggs, and take out all the Yolks
with a Spoon, lay them upon a Plate, and take
great Care not to break any; then beat the Whites
very well, and boil a Quarter of a Pound of Rice in
Water till it is tender; then mix the Rice and
Whites together, ſeaſon it with Nutmeg and Salt:
Greaſe a Cloth with Butter, and pour this into the
Cloth, then boil it an Hour: In the mean Time,
take a clean Frying-pan and a thick Slice of Butter
over a quick Fire, make the Butter brown; then
put in the Yolks and fry them whole, turning each
ſeparate very carefully; then add to them a Jill of
Water, two Spoonfuls of Catchup, one of Walnut
Pickle, and toſs it up, pour it on the Diſh, and throw
the Balls over it; take the Whites out of the Cloth,
and cut into thin Slices, and lay round them. Garniſh the Diſh with fried Parſley.

To ragoo Eggs.

BEAT ten Eggs, and take the Crumb of a Penny
French Roll ſoak'd in Cream, and mix it well
with the Eggs, add green Thyme, Sweet-marjoram,
and Parſley cut ſmall, Nutmeg, Mace, Pepper and
Salt,

Salt, boil this in a Calf's Bladder; take a Pint of fresh Mushroom-buttons, and fry them brown in Butter, add to them a Pint of fresh Water, and boil half a Hundred Asparagus, cut off the tender Part of the Tops into Half-inch Lengths, and stew amongst the Mushrooms, add Walnut Pickle and Verjuice of each a Spoonful, let it boil till the Liquor is half consumed; then thicken it with half a Jill of plain Butter-sauce, and take the great Egg out of the Bladder, cut it down the Middle, and lay the one Half in the Middle of the Dish; cut the other Half in two, and lay on each Side, pour the Ragoo all over them. Garnish with Sippets, Barberry-berries and Capers.

Plumb Pottage.

TAKE two Houghs of a Bullock, break and put them into a Pot and fill it with Water, and when it boils skim it well, add Thyme and Sweet-marjoram, Cloves, Nutmeg, Pepper and Salt; so let it boil, close covered, till it is a strong Soop: Then take up the Houghs, whose Sinews will be as tender as Marrow, strain the Soop into an Earthen-pot and let it stand to cool; then take off all the Fat and put the Soop into a large Hash-pan, grate the Crumb of a Two-penny Loaf and add to it, sweeten it with Sugar to your Taste; then take two Pounds of the best Raisins, a Pound of Prunes, and a Pound of Currants, boil them in the Soop a Quarter of an Hour, and so send it up.

To make Pork Sausages.

TAKE a Hind-chine of Pork, skin it and shred it very fine, as above directed; season it with Pepper, Salt, and dried Sage, mix it well, and when it is beat fine fill your Skins, and they will keep as long as Beef Sausages. But all Sausages are to be put into the smallest Skins, Sheeps Guts are fittest for them; but if you cannot get Sheep Skins, the smallest of the Beef or Hog Skins, which must not be filled above half full.

To

To make Saufages *without Guts.*

TAKE a Pound of lean Mutton, and a Quarter of a Pound of Beef-fuet fhred very fmall, and beat it in a Mortar to a fine Pafte, feafon it with *Jamaica* and Black-pepper, Nutmeg, Salt, Thyme, Sweet-marjoram and Parfley; then drudge Flour on the Table, and roll the Saufage with your Hands into Rolls the Thicknefs of Saufages, and make them into various Shapes, as O, S, C, X, or in any other Shape as your Fancy directs: And when you have Turkey-pouts or Chickens roafted or boiled, lay thefe Saufages on a Tin-pan and fet them in a quick Oven, or before the Fire and broil them, and lay round and over the Fowl or Fowls, with Gravy on the Difh.

To ftew Pigeons.

PLUCK and finge the Pigeons clean, and wafh them, ftuff their Crops with Force-meat, cut off their Legs and turn up their Thighs, put under the Wings as for baking; then put them into a Stew-pan, and cover them with Water, fet them on a flow Stove clofe covered, and let them ftew till they are tender, turning and skimming them often; when their Liquor is almoft confumed, add to it a Pint of Veal-gravy, Force-meat Balls, and Catchup, let them ftew till there is but what is fufficient for Sauce; then add to it a Spoonful of pickled Mufh-rooms, a Spoonful of Walnut Pickle, a little Butter, and tofs all together: Lay Rafhers of Bacon all over them on the Difh. Garnifh with Lemon and green Parfley.

A Sham Pig.

BOIL and peal as many Potatoes as will be the Bulk of a little Pig, which you muft take while they are hot, and beat a Quarter of a Pound of Butter in them, break fix Eggs (leaving out the Whites
of

of four) very well, and mix with the Potatoes; add to them Sugar, Nutmeg and Salt, to your Taſte; let them ſtand to cool, and then make it up in the Form of a roaſted Pig; make a Skin to cover it of Paſte as for a ſtanding Pye; let it have Head, Ears, and Mouth in the Form of a roaſted Pig; let it be ſet in an Oven and baked brown: Then take a little clarified Butter, and a few clean Feathers, dip their Ends in the Butter, and whisk all the Pig with it, juſt as it is taken out of the Oven; this will make the Paſte ſhine as a natural Pig's Skin. For Sauce, have melted Butter, Sugar and red Wine, then ſerve it up.

A Sham Turkey.

TAKE half a Pound of Butter and a Jill of ſweet Cream, boil it till the Butter is melted, then take two Pounds of Flour, add a grated Nutmeg, a little Sugar and Salt, and pour your Cream and boiled Butter into the Flour, and make it into a Paſte. Pick and waſh clean half a Pound of Currants, ſtone and cut ſmall a Quarter of a Pound of Raſins, cut an Ounce of Orange-peel very ſmall, and work all into this Paſte, making it up in the Form of a boiled Turkey; take a Sheet of Puff-paſte and lay over the Breaſt, Wings and Thighs, as the natural Shape of a Turkey, ſet it on a flat-bottomed Diſh, and bake it in a ſlow Oven an Hour; make ſome Balls of Puff-paſte and bake them; lay boiled Rice round the Diſh; and for Sauce, plain melted Butter, ſweeten'd with Sugar and two Spoonfuls of Rheniſh; ſet this Turkey on the Diſh, pour the Sauce round, and the Balls, ſo ſerve it up.

N. B. If the Reader is a good Mechanick, may with the above, ſham any Sort of Wild or Tame-fowl, and it may perhaps be a great Diſappointment to Gormandizers, and a very agreeable one to others.

<i>To make</i> Sauſages <i>of</i> Beef.

TAKE two Pounds of the Inſide of a Surloin of Beef, and half a Pound of Beef-ſuet cut very ſmall on a Shreading-board; add <i>Jamaica</i> and Black-pepper, Salt, Sweet-marjoram, and Thyme; beat this well in a Marble Mortar, with half a Jill of Red-wine or old Beer; then fill the Guts, and hang them in the Kitchen: When they are to be uſed broil them on the Cranks, with two Spoonfuls of Water in a Plate or Tin-pan under them, to intermix with their Gravy.

<i>To make</i> Sauſages <i>of</i> Mutton.

TAKE a Loin of fat Mutton, skin it and take out all the Sinews, ſhred the Fat and Lean very ſmall on a Shreading-board; add half a Jill of Water to it, and ſeaſon with <i>Jamaica</i> and Black-pepper; the ſmall Skins to be filled for preſent Uſe, and broil them as above directed.

<i>To make</i> Puff-paſte.

MIX the Flour with cold Water, and weigh the Paſte; to every Pound of Paſte put half a Pound of Butter, roll out the Paſte and divide the Butter into three Parts, laying one Part on each Sheet, throwing Flour on every Time, and roll it three Times after all the Butter is laid on; if it is froſty, mix the Flour with Water Milk-warm.

P. S. Be ſure to roll the Paſte 'till all the Butter is well mixed, or it will run out in the baking. This Paſte is for Puddings, Paſties, Diſh-pyes, Florentines, or Minced-pyes.

Paſte <i>for ſtanding</i> Cruſts.

TO ſeven Pounds of Flour take three Pounds of Butter and three Pints of Water, boil the Butter and Water till it is melted, then skim off the Butter and

and mix it with Flour, likewiſe the remaining Flour with Water, and the Paſte all together with your Hands; when it is well mixed, cut the Paſte into little Pieces and lay on the Table to cool; then work them all together, and raiſe it into a Pye or Pyes.

Another Paſte *for ſtanding* Cruſts.

TAKE ſome Beef or Sheep-ſuet, which cut ſmall and put into a Braſs-pan, ſet it on a clear Fire at a good Diſtance, if it ſtands over hot it's in Danger of burning the Fat; and when it is diſcharged, take it off the Fire, and drain all the Fat into a Sieve, letting it run into a clean broad Earthen-pot; when it is cold, to a Pound of this Fat take a Pint of Milk, a little Salt, and boil and mix it with the Flour as above: This makes a much better Cruſt in Winter, when Butter is ſtrong, than Butter does. There are few Criticks can diſcover the Taſte of the Fat, for the Milk diverts it, and likewiſe hinders the Paſte from cracking.

Lent *minced* Pyes.

TAKE a Pound of Apple-pulp, half a Pound of Lemon-peel cut ſmall, half a Pound of hard boiled Yolks of Eggs chopped ſmall, and a Pound of Currants clean picked and waſhed, half a Pound of Raiſins ſtoned and cut ſmall, with half a Pound of Sugar; mix all together, and bake it with Puff-paſte in Pans, or in ſtanding Cruſts.

Another Way for Faſt *minced* Pyes.

TAKE a Pound of boiled Potatoes, beat into it a Pound of ſweet Butter, with a Pound of Apple-pulp; alſo Mace, Cinnamon, Cloves, and Nutmeg pounded, half a Pound of Sugar, a Pound and a Half of Currants, a Pound of Raiſins ſtoned and cut ſmall, and half a Jill of Sack; mix them well together, and bake it as above.

4

Another Sort of minced Pyes.

TAKE a Pound of Calf's Feet ſhred very ſmall, with two Pounds of Beef-ſuet, but all the Skin muſt be taken from it; add two Pounds of Currants clean picked and waſhed, aPound of Prunes ſcalded, ſtoned and cut ſmall, half a Pound of Apple-pulp, a Pound of Almonds blanched and beat to a Paſte, half a Pound of Lemon-peel cut ſmall, half a Pound of moiſt Sugar, of Red-wine and Sack each half a Jill: Seaſon to your Taſte with an equal Quantity of Cinnamon, Mace, Nutmeg, and Cloves; mix all well together, and bake as you knead the Pyes.

Another Way to make minced Pyes.

TAKE a Pound of the fatteſt of Beef, and two Pounds of the Kidney-ſuet, ſhred them together till both are ſo ſmall as you cannot perceive the leaſt Bit of the Beef, only it gives a carnation Colour to the Suet; then add two Pounds of well picked Currants, a Pound of ſtoned Raiſins, and half a Pound of Prunes ſcalded, ſtoned, and cut ſmall with the Raiſins; ſeaſon with the above-named Seaſonings: Alſo the Wine, Sack, and the above Quantity of Sugar, with four Ounces of Lemon, and three Ounces of Citron-peel cut ſmall, and to be all well mixed together.

A Trennill Pye.

TAKE a Trennill of a good fat Calf, open and waſh it in many Waters very clean, let it lie all Night in Salt, and boil it till it's tender; then ſhred it as ſmall as minced Pye-meat, and ſeaſon it with *Jamaica*-pepper and Salt; take Prunes, Raiſins, Currants, and Sugar, of each half a Pound; pick the Currants, ſtone the Raiſins and Prunes, cut and mix them all together. They that will be thrifty, may ſkim the Trinnill well in Time of boiling, and it will diſcharge as much Fat as will make a ſtanding Cruſt for it, inſtead of Butter; and if cleanly done, it will be as ſweet as Butter. *How*

How to dry Plumbs.

TAKE large white *magnum bonum* Plumbs; and to every Pound of Plumbs take two Pounds of Sugar; and to every Pound of Sugar add a Pint of hard Water, and boil it ten Minutes: Rub every Plumb with a clean Cloth, and put them into an Earthen flat-bottomed Mug; pour over them the boiling Syrup, and, cover it with Paper cloſe, let them ſtand twenty-four Hours; then take the Syrup from them, and boil it a Quarter of an Hour: In which Time, take the Skin off the Plumbs, and ſet each Plumb upon its End with the Stalk uppermoſt; and when the Syrup hath boiled the above Time, pour it upon the Plumbs, and ſo repeat it ſix Times in the above Manner; then let them ſtand a Week without boiling the Syrup, and then boil it till it is ropey, pour it on the Plumbs, let them ſtand three Weeks, then boil the Syrup again; and let them ſtand a Month, in which Time they will have a ſoft Candy; then take them out of the Pot, and lay them on an Earthen-diſh, and ſift a little double-refined Sugar over them: Let them dry in the Sun or before a Fire, and ſo keep them for Uſe.

How to make Wormwood Drops.

BEAT the Whites of two new laid Eggs on a Pewter-plate with the Back of a Caſe-knife, till the Froth is ſo ſtiff, that you may cut it into Parcels; then beat and ſift through a Tiffany-ſieve a Pound of double-refined Sugar, which beat with the Eggs, add a Spoonful of Orange-flour Water, and beat it to the Stiffneſs of light Paſte; then drop on it three Drops of the Oil of Wormwood, and mix it well: Lay a little of this on a ſquare Pane of Glaſs, or a *Holland* glazed Brick, powder a Pennyworth of Cocheneal, and mix with the Bulk of an Egg of this beat-up Mixture, and marble the other with the red Colour; but you muſt mix it ſo as to make the White and Red tranſparent. Drop them upon

glazed

glazed Paper, that is, white Paper glazed with a Sleek-ſtone; let not each be above the Size of a Filberd, and ſet them in the Sun or before a Fire to dry. Put them on clean Paper into a Paper-box, and keep them for Uſe.

To make Lemon Drops.

PARE the yellow Skin of a freſh Lemon, cut it ſmall, and put it into a Quarter of a Jill of the beſt Brandy, let it ſtand twelve Hours; then take the Whites of two new-laid Eggs, and mix with the ſame Quantity of double-refined Sugar, beat and ſifted as in the above Manner: When it is done, beat into it a Spoonful of the Brandy that the Lemon Skin lay in, mix it well, and dry them as above; then drop it on glazed Paper, and dry it as before directed. Box them up, and keep them for Uſe.

To make Jumballs.

INFUSE an Ounce of Gum-arabick, put to it a large Wine-glaſs of Orange-flour Water, the ſame Quantity of Roſe-water, and let them ſtand twenty-four Hours; then take the Whites of three freſh Eggs, with a Pound and a Half of double-refined Sugar ſifted, beat them to a Stiffneſs; then take the Gum, which muſt be as thick as clear boiled Starch, beat it with the Eggs, blanch and beat two Ounces of *Jourdon* Almonds, with a Spoonful of Roſe-water, and the above Ingredients all to a fine Paſte: Then roll it into Balls and flatten them a little, lay them on glazed Paper and Wires, and ſet them in an Oven to bake; when they are enough, keep them for Uſe.

To make Currant-paſte.

TAKE two Quarts of pick'd ripe Red-currants, and put them into Jars, cover them cloſe and ſet them into an Oven two Hours; then ſtrain them through a Flannel-bag, and take two Pounds of Loaf-ſugar, wet it in Water and boil it to a Candy-height; then put to it a Pint of the Currant Juice, but don't let it boil after it is in, ſtir it well together, and put it into an Earthen-mug till the next Day; then drop it in little Cakes on Wafer-paper, and dry it in the Sun, or in a very cool Oven.

Marmalade *of* Orange.

BOIL twelve thin skin'd *Seville* Oranges, that is freſh, three Times, removing them out of the boiling Pot each Time, till they are ſo tender that a Straw will run through them; then take them out, and to every Pound of Oranges take two Pounds of double-refined Sugar, to every Pound of Sugar add half a Pint of Water, and boil it in a clean Braſs-pan on a clear Stove: In the mean Time, cut each Orange, and take out the Inſides (take Care of the Juice and Meat) and Seeds; cut the Orange Skins into very thin Slices, and put into the boiling Sugar, let it boil till the Skins are clear, keep ſtirring it; then put all the Inſides into the Marmalade, and boil it till it begins to ſpark and fly, but be ſure to keep it ſtirring all the Time; ſo put it into Glaſſes or Jelly-pots, laying white Paper over it dipped in Brandy, and tie over it Bladders; then keep it for Uſe.

To preſerve Oranges *whole.*

TAKE ſix of the beautifulleſt large *Seville* O-ranges to be got, and lay them in Salt and Water three Days; then boil them in Water, and ſhift them as above; and when they are ſo tender that a Straw will run through them, take them out and cut a round Piece off each Top of the Oranges, not to exceed the Breadth of a Shilling, and with a Tea-ſpoon take out all the Seeds, but none of the Meat; then take ſix Pounds of double-refined Su-gar, put to it two Quarts of Water, and boil it ten Minutes; ſet each Orange on its End in a flat-bot-tomed

tomed Pot, and put within them the round Piece you cut out; then pour upon them the boiling Syrup, and lay a Delf-plate over to keep them down. Thus boil it once every Day for 12 Times, after put each Orange into a Gally-pot juſt fit for it, to be covered with Syrup, and tie a Bladder over each Pot, ſo keep them for Uſe.

How to make Orange Chips.

TAKE the freſh Skin of *Seville* Oranges, whoſe Juice has been uſed for Punch, and lay them in Salt and Water three Days; then boil them tender, ſhifting them as above, and take out all the Strings of the Inſides; put them into an Earthen-pot, make a Syrup of common Lump-ſugar, and boil it three Times a Week the firſt Fortnight; then let it ſtand a Month longer, and take the Skins out of the Syrup and waſh them in clear Water, turn them down on a Sieve, and ſo dry them in a ſlow Oven; then cut them into Chips, and according to the Quantity, if three Pounds of Chips, two Pounds of Sugar, wet it with Water and boil it Candy-height; then put in your Chips and let them boil, dip a Slice into the Syrup and blow it through, if it flies like Snow, you muſt take them out and ſpread them on an Earthen-diſh to cool, ſo keep them for Uſe.

Red Marmalade of Quinces.

PARE, core and ſlice your Quinces, and to every Pound of Quinces take a Pound and a Half of Loaf-ſugar, and to each Pound of Sugar a Jill of Water; ſet them on a Stove in a clean Pan, and heat all together ſlowly till it comes to a red Colour; then ſharpen the Fire, boil it to a ſtiff Gelly, and pot it for Uſe.

To make *white* Marmalade *of* Quinces.

PARE and quarter your Quinces, and have ready
a Pan, to every Pound of Quinces take a Pound
and a half of double-refined Sugar, wet with fair
Water; put your fliced Quinces into boiling Water, and boil the Sugar Candy-height; when the
Quinces are tender, drain the Water from them thro'
a Hair-fieve, put it into the Sugar, and let all boil
till the Quinces be clear; then put it into Pots or
Glaffes for Ufe.

To make Rasberry Cakes.

TO every Pound of Rasberries take a Pound of
double-refined Sugar, mix and put into a Pre-
ferving-pan; boil it on a clear Stove, keep it ftirring all the Time, let it boil till it is a thick ftrong
Stiffnefs, and fet it by till it is cold; then make it
into little Cakes, lay them on a Paper to dry, and
keep them for Ufe.

To dry red Currants *in* Strops.

PICK out all the Seeds of the Currants on the
Stalks, boil Leaf-fugar Candy-height, and put
in your Currants; boil and take them out Stalk
by Stalk, and lay them on a large Stone-difh feparate
to cool; duft grated double-refined Sugar, and turn
them every Day till they are dry: So box them up
for Ufe.

To make Gingerbread.

TAKE four Pounds of Treacle into a Pan, and
fet it on a clear Fire till it is fcalding hot;
then ftir into it half a Pound of Sweet-butter and a
Jill of Brandy, and pour it into a Bowl; add to it
two Ounces of beat Ginger, the fame Quantity of
powdered *Jamaica* Pepper, an Ounce of Coriander
Seeds, the fame of Carraway Seeds, all well beat,
and

and beat four Pounds of Flour into it very well; when the Lumps are very well beat out, cut half a Pound of Lemon-peal into long Pieces, greaſe a large Cake-pan with Butter, and divide it into four Loaves, laying the fourth Part of the Lemon-peal on each Lair: It will take ſix Hours baking.

The *Cordial Hunters* Gingerbread.

TAKE three Pints of red Port, and four Pounds of Loaf-ſugar; boil them in a broad Braſs-pan, let it boil till it is a Syrup, and take it off the Fire; add to it a Pint of Brandy, Cinamon, Race Ginger, Mace, Cloves, and Nutmeg, of each half an Ounce finely beat to a Powder, grated Manſhot Bread dried in an Oven or before the Fire four Pounds, three of which put to the above Ingredients, and boil it till it is thick; then let it cool, work up the other Pound of dry grated Bread, and make it into various Shapes, as Prints, ſmall Rolls, and little Cakes: Lay it on white Paper to dry, and keep it for Uſe. A ſmall Piece of this is a Dram in the Morning.

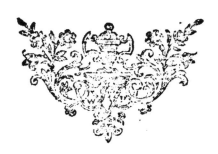

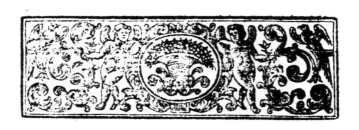

INDEX.

INDEX.

To

INDEX.

To

INDEX.

Z   A

I N D E X.

A

INDEX.

To

I N D E X.

To

I N D E X.

Veal

I N D E X.

F I N I S.

I N D E X

TO THE

A P P E N D I X.

A a   *To*

A

A

P L A N

O F

HOUSE-KEEPING.

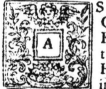

S complete Housewifery ornaments a
Queen, so does it every Lady in the
Kingdom that possesses that Treasure;
the Value of which preserves both
Health and Fortune: She will not be
imposed upon by extravagant Servants,
as she well knows what the daily Expence of her
House amounts to: Neither by Indolence, for she
can see into that by surveying her House wherein
that Decorum and Oeconomy shines illustriously; if
humane, her Servants will love, fear, and obey her:
But this may not be the Case of the young unexperienced Lady whose Housekeeper is deputed Mistress,
who perhaps may fancy herself supreme, and take as
much State and Attendance upon her as the Lady
herself can do; for vain Glory is a great Prompter
where Integrity and Judgment is wanting, by which
great Fortunes have been impaired, either unjustly,
carelesly, or extravagantly. The Courage of one
Cook who served a wealthy Esquire in this Neighbourhood, gave the Lady's Maid the Mortification
of seeing her take a large Sauce-pan full of Butter,
that

that she for want of Judgment oiled in melting for Sauce, and tossed it into the Sink that she put her dirty Water in to run into the Venal: The Lady's Maid telling one of the Servants of the Waste, was answered, That she did frequently tofs her oil'd Butter into that Sink, and this she aver'd to me, that the least Quantity of Butter could not be less than one Pound and a Half at that one Time; yet this Lady's Maid, although she was a Relation to her Mistress, had not the Courage to reprove the Cook, nor durst tell the Housekeeper, left she should ask her, what was her Businefs in the Kitchen? or call her Spy-teller, Magpy; or give Orders to the Cook to befpatter her with a Ladle full of Fat whenever she came into her Territories.

Such Hazards attends those that dare oppose extravagant Cooks, or indolent Housekeepers that are Strangers to every Thing worthy of Praise, and consequently very dangerous Kitchen Officers, for they confume their Masters Substance unmercifully: Had she tofs'd this oiled Butter into an Earthen-pot, it might have fried Fish, Fritters, or Pancakes, covered potted Fowls, Beef, or Fish; but tossing it into the Venal, is a Crime that deserves the Punishment of Hunger, and Bitternefs of the Want of Butter all her Days. That is, after she had left her Plenty, and returned to her primative homely Cottage, as wilful Waste brings woful Want; for which Reafon the good and profitable Servant is on the fafeft Side: She that holds fast her Integrity, and would do her Duty to the best of her Knowledge, thefe Refolutions deferves Improvement.

As I have acted in the Station of Cook and Housekeeper, fo have I been very fuccefsful in pleasing the Families I served in that Station; and as I have a great Regard for the worthy Sort of thefe Servants, *and*

and would take a great Pleasure to improve thefe
Worthies; that is, by telling them how I difcharg'd
the Truft of Deputy. I made the following Refolutions, and kept them, refolved to do Juftice to
Mafters and Servants; not to leave that to be done
in the Morning that ought to have been done at
Night; refolved not to wafte nor confume the Property of my Mafter, nor fuffer any of his Servants
to wrong him to my Knowledge; refolved to be as
careful of every Individual of my Truft, as if the
Fortune had been my own; refolved to rife early in
the Morning, and never to exceed Six o'Clock if I
was in Health, nor to grudge rifing two Hours
fooner if I had an elegant Dinner to fend up; refolved that every Servant fhould have their Meat in due
Seafon, and likewife every Fowl that was fed for
my Mafter's Table. My great Care was to keep
the feathered Flock clear of Difeafes, which, without great Care and Pains they are very fubject to;
and to prevent Diftempers, I never bought Chickens
with their Feet tied together, and ftopped into Baf-
kets and Creels, for this Reafon: The Birds are con-
fined to lie on their Sides, which the ftepping or
trotting of the Horfes makes them full of Bruifes,
and puts them into Fevers: But the prudent Farmers does not ufe their feathered Flock fo, they
have large Creels or Baskets, puts them loofe in,
lets them have Room to ftand upon their Feet, and
they are no worfe for their Journey; thefe were the
Birds I always chufed to buy, and as my Chicken
Coops had Partitions that took out to make them
lefs or bigger Appartments, I always kept each Brood
to themfelves, for as foon as mixt with Strangers
Battle-arrays enfued, which, to prevent I never mixt
them after: I have found by Reafon of their Battles
their Heads have been fo fore, that they could not
feed; nay, the Conquerors got Bruifes with their
Wings flapping in the Coops with the battling:
Yet the Brood that is hatched and brought up together

gether feeds fat, and quarrels none. Every Night their Troughs were washed clean, and clean Hay put under them at Six o'Clock in the Morning; Barley-meal mixt pretty stiff with boiling Water, and when cool dipped into skim'd Milk, and so given the Chickens in their clean Troughs: My Turkey Pouts and Capons I found fed best at their Liberty loose in a House; I made them Crammings of the same I fed the Chickens with every Morning, having their House clean swept, and clean Straw laid in a Corner to rub themselves in, which is as refreshing to them as their Meat, and when they were full took the Meat from them, served them at Twelve, and again at Six in the Evening, took the Meat from the Chickens, and served them as above.

My green Geese and Ducks fed best together in a House loose; then I fed them either with ground Malt and Butter-milk, or unground Malt with boiling Water poured over it, the last Thing at Night: This feeds Chickens fat, giving it them in the above Manner; yet I don't think it feeds Chickens, Turkeys, or Capons so white as Milk and Barley-meal does, but as fat it will feed them. I drove them once a Week to a Pond to wash themselves, which gave them a great Pleasure; they would flap their Wings, and rejoice when they returned amongst their clean Straw.

I never grudged the Pains I took in feeding the Fowls, for when I sent them up to the Master's Table, they were received with Pleasure and Applause; that sufficiently rewarded my Labour; yet it was no more than my Duty, and what every Servant in that Post ought to do, or see it done. A new married Lady related to my Mistress, who had a lingering Illness, occasioned by a Miscarriage of her first Child, was persuaded by her Husband, to take an airing with him in the Coach, and to dine with my Mistress; he he ordering a Servant to let her know his Intention, and that there might be a boiled Chicken for his Wife; so I had Orders for four boiled Chickens, two young Ducks, and two Turkey Pouts roasted: At the Hour appointed the Esquire and his Lady came, and Dinner being ready, was sent up, and met with a most grateful Reception from this worthy Esquire, who, with Admiration beheld his Lady eat up a whole Chicken; who said to her, Much Good may it do you, my Dear, for I am sure you have not eat so hearty a Meal this two Months: It is very true, Sir, answered she, and the Reason is, that I never see such a Chicken in my own House, for it is no bigger than a Partridge, and as fat as a Quail, so beautifully white, quite different from my Chickens at Home, that are Skeletons, and of a different Hue and Taste from this Chicken, that seems to sit very easy on my Stomach. I have had a boiled Chicken every Day to my Dinner these six Weeks, but not one like this; nor did I ever see a fat Fowl at my Table, which I impute to improper feeding. In all Probability that must be the Reason, answered my Mistress, for I have very often taken Notice of your Poultry at the Table, and am very sure that if they were duly attended, and proper Care taken of them, they would be fat, and they are not fit to eat otherwise. So I have experienced, replied the other Lady, yet the only Reason that I can give, is, that my Cook was trained at *London,* where she had all her Fowls fed and kill'd ready for cooking: She is the only grave Servant that I have, and was well recommended; I am therefore unwilling to accuse her for a Fault that I cannot give a proper Direction to amend, so unexperienced a Housekeeper am I, that was left an Orphan, and married just out of the Boarding-school, for which Reason my Health and Fortune may be impaired, and I utterly unable to rectify it. My dear, despairing Cousin, answered my Mistress, pluck up your Spirits,

and

and there will be no Hazard of Health and Fortune,
for you shall stay with me, and try the Sovereign
Virtue of my Kitchen Physick; for in my Opinion,
that is the only Medicine you want at present; and
I will send my Cook to give yours a Lesson of her
Method of feeding Poultry, and many Things that
may differ from what she has been acquainted with:
That is, to shew her how much more is required
of the Country Cooks, than there is of the City
Cooks; and, added she, I am very sure that she will
be ready and willing to give her wholesome Cookery Advice. Then, answered she, I will be infinitely
obliged to her, and if you can spare her she may go
in the Coach which is returning Home, for I am
fully determined to try the Virtue of your Kitchen
Physick. You oblige me much my dear Cousin.

So my Lady came and told, that there must be
some Need of my Advice to feed their Poultry, and
if she be sociable, help her in her Deficiencies; if
not, give yourself no Concern but come Home in
the Morning according to my Directions.

I went, and was kindly received by my Sister
Cook; the Lady's Maid went to wait on her Mistress, and there was none to interrupt our Conversation: So having our Tea brought in great Order,
she dismissed the Footman, and said, Statesmen have
private Interviews in Politicks, Merchants in Com-
merc, so let ours be upon the Art of Cookery. I answered, If that be our Talent, let us be profitable Servants, and improve it. Then said she, If I improve I
must be the Beggar. I answered, If there was any Knowledge in my Possession worth Acceptance she might
command it. Then, said she, my greatest Want is to
know how to make Fowls fat; as in the Town I
had them fed, plotted, and ready for the Pot or
Spit: But here I have them to feed, and instead
of making them fat, behold, they are all Skeletons,
and

and more dies in the Coops than lives: Chickens, Turkey Pouts, young Ducks, and green Geese dies, or pines in the Coops. Indeed Sister, said I, where there is so much Sickness in the Coops, it may endanger the Family's Healths in the House. Sickness amongst Poultry, do you say, then I am a very improper Physician; nor will pretend the least Skill in curing their Sickness: It must be Sickness that causes so great a Mortality in the Coops, but this I imputed to their quarrelling; and more especially amongst the Chickens, which I thought killed one another, said she, or rather wounded and bruised each other. Answered I, the Agony of which might bring Fevers upon the wounded, that might occasion their Deaths; and likewise infect the Conquerors, and the whole feathered Flock. But how to prevent it, said she, let me know; for Judgment may be wanting, but Care and Pains was not: For every Morning I see all the Drawers that receive their Dung taken out, their Troughs clean washed, and fresh Meat made them at the same Time; which Meat stood by them, to eat when they pleased, till the next Morning, when they were served again: Nor did I let any of the dead lie in the Coop any Time, lest they should stink, and so offend the others.

Indeed, Sister, answered I, I never understood whether the Poultry have the Sense of smelling, as they have no Noses; yet I am very well assur'd, that Cleanliness is a great Help to their thriving: But letting Meat stand perpetually before them must pall their Appetites; they are delicate Creatures, and loath their Meat when satisfied, so that I never fail to take it from them in ten Minutes after I have served them, a sufficient Time to fill themselves in: As to Quarrels, I never have any amongst my Chickens, for this Reason, having a separate Partition for every separate Brood, and this keeps Peace; but
inter-

intermixing them with Strangers is bloody Wars:
Every Morning they have clean Hay laid under them,
and every Day thrice fed, at Six in the Morning, at
Twelve, and at Six in the Evening: Their Troughs
are washed clean, and as much Meal mixt in the
Morning as will serve them all Day. Turkeys and
Capons I feed in a House by themselves, on the same
Meat I feed the Chickens with, only I roll it up in
Crammings, and lets them Sweet-milk to drink.
My Ducks and green Geese I feed loose in a House,
with ground Malt and Butter-milk, or scalds Malt:
Now I can prove by my Book of Poultry, both in
the Poultry living, and Poultry killed for the Family's Use, that I have been accountable to my Lady
of every individual Fowl, even to the smallest Chick-
en. Then certainly I must have been a very unpro-
fitable Servant, answered she, for I have not only
wasted the Property of my Master, but am terribly
afraid I have impaired the Health of his Lady, by
sending her up Chickens that were not fit to eat:
For when I consider the Difference betwixt the Chickens I bought of the Poulterers, and those I fed, and
sent that dear Lady to eat, they must have hurt her
delicate Constitution, and to give Pain to so good
a Lady is Sacrilege; or is it possible Ignorance can
make an Attonement for such a Crime? Yes, very
possible, answered I, as it is a common Crime, which
I am afraid many fine Gentry are Sufferers by, and
are fed with distempered Poultry by slothful and indolent Servants; which is not your Case, whose Industry and Integrity is firm, but Judgment was
wanting in Poultry feeding, which made it a Misfortune, but no Crime.

As for Turkeys, Capons, Chickens, Ducks, and
Geese, clean your Coups of them; let the Ducks and
green Geese be put into a Pasture where there is Water for to wash in, and feed them with Corn thrice a
Day; let the other Poultry at Liberty, and feed them,
but

but you muſt expect Death for moſt of them. Then
let your Maid clean all the Coops and Houſes,
buy in a freſh Stock, and get acquainted with the
Farmers Wives; theſe in ſhort are the beſt Birds
Mothers, for they feed them with the Overplus of
their Milkneſs; nay, they have a Share of their own
Victuals, will fly upon the Tables and pick the Meat
off their Trenchers, theſe are half-fed to your Hand:
Charge the good Wives not to tie their Feet, but
to put them into a large Creel or Basket looſe. Never confine your Turkeys or Capons in Coops, it
cripples and cauſes them to pine inſtead of fatning,
and will ſwarm with Lice for Want of Liberty to
pick their Feathers. Sweep their Houſe every Day,
lay them clean ſtraw, and have the ſame Pleaſure of
your Feathered-flock I have of mine. I will, anſwers
ſhe, purſue this Pleaſure with Diligence and Care,
with a thouſand Thanks to you for the wholeſome
Leſſon you have taught me, for although I gave great
Content in Town, I find myſelf very deficient in
the Country; in Town I made my Market every
Day, the Butchers Meat ſo freſh and ſweet that my
Beef-gravy made Sauces, and Soops delicious: But
here we kill a Beef once a Month, and that alters
the Caſe, for I can but have freſh Beef one Week
in the whole Month; ſo there is three Weeks of
the Month I have no Beef-ſoop nor Beef-gravy for
Sauces, without ſending to the Market for freſh Beef.

As ſalt Beef is not fit for Soops or Sauſes to be
ſure, but if I have plenty of freſh Beef, I can make
Gravy that will keep two Months as ſtrong and as
delicious as the firſt Day; and if you will try the
Experiment when you kill a Beef, take the four
Houghs and break them, ſeaſon with a little Salt,
Jamaica and Black-pepper; then pack them down
in a large Stewing-pot, with a Quart of Water,
and cover the Pot cloſe with Paſte: Cut and ſeaſon
the Beef's Neck in the above Manner, pot and paſte
it

·it alſo, and heat an Oven as hot as for baking Houſhold Bread; then ſet in theſe Pots, daub up your Oven,
and let them ſtand all Night: In the Morning take
them out, and the Sinews will be as tender ſtew'd
as Marrow; which Sinews take from the other Meat,
cut them into half Inch-lengths, and put them ſeparate into Earthen-pots, about the Size or rather
larger than a Jill; then ſtrain the Gravy through a
clean Hair-ſieve: Take up the two Necks of Beef,
ſtrain the Gravy all into one Pot, skim off all the
Fat, and ſtrain the Gravy through a clean Flannel
Bag; then take a well tinned Soop-pan, ſet it upon a clear Stove of Cinders, put in this ſtrong Gravy,
boil it quickly half an Hour, and cover the potted
Sinews with it: Have as many Pint broad Earthen-
pots as will hold the Remainder of the Gravy, leave
Room for half an Inch deep of the Beef-fat that you
skimmed off the Gravy, which Fat boil up in a Sauce-
pan, pour it boiling hot over each Pot of Gravy,
and let it ſtand till it be thoroughly cold; the Gravy
will be a ſtiff Gelly, and the Sinews will anſwer
Soops or Ragoos. The ſame of Pallates.—So there
is Gravy for Soops or Sauces, much ſtronger than
you can pretend to make by frying the Beef, and
after boiling it is always ready and ſaves much Trouble: I never want a Store by me, for I can by boiling it to a fine Glue, keep it ſix Months, with cloſe
ſealing in little Pots; and if a Meſs of Soop is wanted, I have it in a Minute.

Neither do I ever want Chicken Broth, for when
I have boiled Chickens, I pack them cloſe in a Pan
that juſt holds them, and this makes their Broth
ſtronger; then I take the Bones of a Leg of Veal,
and the Griſſel of the Knockle, breaks and waſhes
them clean, ſo puts my Chicken Broth into a little
Stewing-pot, with the Veal Bones, two or three
Blades of Mace, and paſtes the Pot cloſe down, ſo
ſets it in an Oven all Night, skims off all the Fat
in

in the Morning, and puts the Broth through a clean
Flannel Bag; then boils this strong Chicken Broth
to a strong Gelly, puts it into small Earthen-cups,
and covers it with the Fat I skimmed off: This answers various Uses, for if any of the Family wants
Chichen Broth, I have it for them; or if I want
Gravy for white Sauces, it is ready for my Use. By
this Forecast I save my Master many a Chicken, and
myself the Trouble of killing them.

For the future this Lesson which your have so
frankly given me, answered she, shall be my greatest
Pleasure to practise; for every Word you have spoken
to me convinces me of my Errors, and of the Truth,
Justice, Reason, and Consideration that appertains
to the true Art of Cookery, which I find I have
been prodigious ignorant and deficient in.

Well, says I, as I am the elder Sister, I must except of the Compliment you make me, so let us
sleep on it this Night, and we will rise in the Morning, for I will be on Horseback at Six, Home at
Eight, so to work in the Kitchen at Nine.—At half
an Hour after Five, when I had got on my Cloaths,
behold in comes my Sister to enquire how I had slept
in a strange Bed: Very well, answered I.—That has
not been my Case, said she, for I have been so tortured with dreaming of sick Poultry all the Night,
that I arose at Four o'Clock, and have set all the
Prisoners at Liberty, much to my Shame go with
me; and I did behold them accordingly, and saw
the lame, maimed, and the blind. Your green Geese
and Ducks may recover in Time, said I, by bathing
and feeding, but very few of your Chickens.—Not
one, answered she, for they shall die in an Hour, and
I will buy in as many healthy ones at my own Expence, after the House and Coops are clean washed.
Don't kill the Turkey Pouts, but turn them to the
Back-yard, and feed them with Corn and Grass,

Phyfick may fet them to rights again, and this Precaution I give you: Likewife, faid I, fee that you never take Notice to your Lady in the leaft of the Sicknefs that has been in the Coops for this Reafon, becaufe it may do her more Harm in thinking than it has done in eating thofe Chickens; and if you duly obferve the Rules that I have prefcribed to you, there never will be Sicknefs amongft your Poultry.—Fear not, anfwered fhe, I have printed each Article on the Table of each Hand, the Execution of which fhall be my greateft Pleafure.

But here is one proper Item that I muft give you, it fuits this prefent Cafe, as you have no fat Chickens, boil Rice in Water, and after in a little Milk, fweeten it with a little brown Sugar, and it will feed them fat in four Days; but let them be fed four Times a Day with this Rice, Milk, and Sugar.

So after we got Breakfaft I took my Leave, and told her I expected my Vifit repaid me the firft Opportunity; fhe promifed fhe would, and I was at Home as the Clock ftruck Eight. My Lady being told that I was come, fent for me, and asked my Opinion of the Houfe-keeper: I anfwered, Madam, I have a very good Opinion of her, for fhe very frankly owned her Deficiency in Poultry-feeding, and with Pleafure and a Heart full of Gratitude, returned me her unfeigned Thanks for the Method of feeding Poultry that I prefcribed her, which fhe acknowledged was more confiftent with Reafon, than the Method fhe had taken in feeding them; and although her Judgment I believe to be very good in other Refpects, yet fhe feemed more defirous of having my Opinion than of giving her own. I believe her to be a Servant of Worth and Integrity, and very deferving of the Truft repofed in her; and it is my Belief, that you will not for the future fee an ill fed Fowl come to her Mafter's Table, for fhe was a-
mongft

mongſt thém at Four o'Clock·this Morning, Induſtery and Care ſhe wants not.—I am pleaſed, anſwered my Lady, with the Account you have given me of her: Did not you invite her to my Houſe?—I did, Madam, and ſhe promiſed me ſhe would the firſt Opportunity.—I will procure an Opportunity by asking her Miſtreſs, for I have a great Veneration for ſuch Servants as you deſcribe her to be.—To prove the Truth, Madam, ſays I, keep her Lady a Week, and if ſhe has not fat Chickens for her Lady, truſt no more to my Skill.

Well then, anſwered my Miſtreſs, to try the Variety of thy Judgment, I will detain the Lady, and have thy Aſſertion proved. So my Lady made the young Couple very merry at Breakfaſt with the Account that I had given her of their Houſe-keeper, and they all conſented to go Home at the Week's End; accordingly they did ſo, and found ſhe had as fat Chickens and as beautiful as mine, to the great Pleaſure of my Lady as well as hers; and from that Time there was an honeſt Friendſhip contraĉted between her and me. There being ſo great an Intimacy betwixt the two Families, the young Lady uſed to bring her in the Coach with herſelf to pay me a Viſit, for they knew the very great Regard we had for each other; for ſhe was generally eſteemed being both the complete Houſewife, and the virtuous humane Creature. If any poor Family in the Neighbourhood were in Diſtreſs, ſhe informed her Lady of their Want, whoſe Pleaſure was to relieve them. This young Creature took great Delight in doing good, gave Medicines to the Poor for moſt Diſorders, and this worthy Servant was always ready to deliver their Complaints, never grudging the Pains ſhe took for the Poor.

I ſoon after removed from that Family twenty Miles diſtant, ſo that our future Correſpondence was by

writing,

writing, till we both enter'd into the Marriage-state, which put us a greater Distance from each other. Sometime after her Marriage, she wrote me a long Letter, wherein she expressed the Happiness she possessed in one of the best of Husbands, that Love and Riches increased every Day; and begged of me to give her an Account of my Situation of Life. I answered hers, and told the great Pleasure I had in her good Fortune, both in the Blessing of a good Husband and Riches, a Reward for her Virtue and good Works; and told her that as the Situation of my Chance had fallen in a publick Way, (Inn-keeping) which had not afforded me that Tranquillity she possessed: I would not go to Particulars, only acquainted her I was in a middling State, some better and many worse. I was answered with a very moving Epistle, desiring a more particular Relation of my Situation; but I considered as it would not be satisfactory, never answered her last Request, so our Correspondence dropt till after the Publication of my Book of Cookery, (which upon perusal I found I had made Omissions of Receipts, but have since supplied these Wants, as a further Service to my Readers). As she possessed an active Soul, I was perfectly assured that in whatever Station of Life she lived, she would improve her Talent. So having a little spare Time the latter End of last Year, I took Post-chaise and made a Tour thirty Miles cross the Country to see my Friend: She was at a Loss at the first Sight to know who I was, till she heard me speak; she said, There is the Voice, but where is the Person? yet got me in her Arms, saluted and gave a hearty Welcome; and as I had dined on the Road, she made Coffee and Tea, and told me her Husband was not to be at Home till next Day. I said, If I have not the Pleasure of his Company I hope to have yours all to myself: Certainly, said she, only the Interruption of my young Brood; and as she thus spake, in comes five beautiful Daughters, the

the eldeſt was juſt thirteen Years of Age, and the youngeſt eight; ſo neat, andtheir Behaviour, as if they had been come Home from a Boarding-ſchool, to pay their Parents a Viſit, every one making a low Curſy as they entered the Room. We having done Tea, they drunk each two Diſhes, the eldeſt waſhed the China and ſet it into the Store-room, which Door opened into the Room we ſat in; ſo ſays I, Is this yourStore-room? let me ſee how you have it furniſhed. You ſhall ſays ſhe. So in we went. Now, ſays ſhe, behold the Rule and Order of an induſtrious and careful Husband, who built me this Conveniency and ſhelfed it round; on that Side is one with five Partitions for bottled Wines, each containing ten Dozen of Bottles; ſo ſaying, ſhe opened the Lids, took out a Bottle of each Wine, and called for five Glaſſes, filling each Glaſs up with the ſeparate Wines: Now, ſaid ſhe, taſte theſe Wines, and give me your Opinion of them; there is *Burgundy*, *French*, red *Port*, *Frontiniack*, and ſweet *Mountain*. So taſting the Wines, which were all as clear as Rock-water, I ſaid, If I had ſeen theſe Wines in a Gentleman's Houſe or any Tavern, they might have paſſed for Foreign, for they are ſtrong and muſt be of a good Age; new Wines are like new Malt Liquor: Theſe Wines are ruff, well flavoured with Age, and has a ſtrong Body, which I am pretty ſure are all of your own making. She ſmiling told me, I was the firſt that ever diſputed their being foreign; for Gentlemen Stewards have proteſted, that better Wines were not in their Maſters Cellars than the Wines they drunk here; but indeed this is a proper Place for the Bottles, it is warm in Winter, and cool in Summer, ſo is the Cellar below, it being vaulted, and all the Wines are ſeven Years old before they are bottled. For as I ſee there is no halting before Cripples, be that as it will, Gratitude obliges me to let you into the Secret of Made-wines, as frankly as you gave me the Secret of Poultry-feeding, which
you

you shall see; I have not forgot by my feathered
Flock, which are beautifully fat: But first survey
my Conveniency, there stands my Wine-press, where
I made my first great Quantity; I pressed the Fruit
in a Cheese Press, put it into the Cloaths, and so
pressed it in the Cheese Fats, in the same Manner
the Cheese is pressed, so set a broad clean Tub to
save the Juice: But my endearing Man got the Di-
mensions of a Wine Press, and made it his dear self;
likewise he made all the Chests for Flour, Oat-meal,
Barley-meal, Groats, and Bran; likewise these Set
of Boxes for my Salves and Drugs, Shelves for my
Salvers, Delf, and China; and opening the Wine
Cellar-door, said, Behold my Stock of Wines: So
numbering the Casks, said I, Your Stock surmounts
any of our Northern 'Squires that I have seen, for
by my Calculation you have eighteen Hogsheads of
Wine in Casks, besides the fifty Dozen of Bottles;
and this is a Quantity that very few Noblemen have
I dare say: But let us go and have some Conversation, for I long to hear some of your History, and
am sure it will give me infinite Pleasure. So we returned to the Parlour again, finding it clean dusted,
a good Fire, bright Irons, and clean Hearth, we sat
ourselves down, and thus she begun her Narrative.

I think I gave you an Account in a Letter of the
ill Fortune of my Mistress's Maid, in a run-away
Welding with the Footman, which my dear Lady
was so good as to express great Concern for her un-
thinking Maid, that had so poorly bestowed herself
on a simple Fellow that could not labour for Bread
for her, nor himself, and 'tis my Opinion, as soon as
Poverty affects them, he will certainly change his
Livery for a red one; but what Opinion have you
of this Match. Indeed, Madam, answered I, if Pride
and vain Glory will make a good Husband, he has
enough of that. Nay, said the dear Lady, her Wisdom is as small as his, and I wish they may both
deceive

deceive me; but I am determined not to have a giddy young Lafs about me again; you fhall be my Maid and Houfe-keeper, fo hire a profefs'd Cook. I anfwered, I had a very good one of my own making; fhe has been a Servant as long as I have, and is not much inferior to myfelf in Cookery; as to the Houfe-keeping, that I perform, but the Cookery I have taught her, and was enquiring for a Place for her, as fhe has a Sifter that was to come in her Place: You bid me choofe my Affiftant when I firft came to my Place, this is the Servant, and I have proved her Integrity. You have obliged me very much, faid the worthy Lady, in teaching me a Cook in your own Way, for I have very often thought your Fatigue too great, to perform the Part of Cook and Houfe-keeper; for which Reafon I wanted gladly to have had you for my own Maid and Houfe-keeper, but was afraid of not getting fo good a Cook, for you pleafed me in my Meat dreffing: I never liked this fliskey Girl that waited on me, for if fhe had brought me a Meffage of any poor Creatures Complaint, I fee her Countenance turn four; and have rebuked her and faid, I wifhed fhe might not have their Complaint, and meet with as little Pity as feemingly fhe fhewed to thofe in Diftrefs.

So thus I anfwered my dear Angel, *Bleffed are the Merciful, for they fhall receive Mercy.* For Madam, if your Eye be good, God forbid that mine be evil, to the Prejudice of my fellow Creatures; for as far as is in my Power I will cheartfully affift them, both in delivering their Complaints to you, and likewife your Relief to them.—Said fhe, Your Perquifites will be better as to my Caftings, and you have the fame Wages; fo there is a Guinea Earneft for your new Place, and if fix Pounds Wages will do for the Cook, let her hire a Kitchen Maid.

This Preferment I told her to her great Joy, and fhe hired her Sifter, fo they lived in Peace, and did
their

their Work to Admiration : No Servants upon Earth
were more happy than we were of a worthy Mafter,
a pious, generous, and charitable Lady, whofe Humanity was fuch, that fhe fed the Hungry, cloathed
the Naked, and was a great Doctrefs to them afflicted with Sicknefs; happy would be the diftreffed, did
every one difcharge their Stewardfhips like this happy Pair, for they delighted in a rural Life. He built
a Houfe for a School, with two Rooms for the
Mafter and his Wife to live in, and put 40 poor
Children to School, 20 Boys and 20 Girls, cloathed
them every Year, were taught to read, write, and
Vulgar Arithmetick: They likewife cloathed 30 poor
old Men and Women with new Shoes, Stockings,
two Shirts, Hat, Coat, Waiftcoat, and Breeches to
the Men; and the Women they gave Shoes, Stockings,
Gown, Petticoat, Apron, Shifts, Caps, &c. And
when they had all got on their new Cloathing, my
good Mafter and Miftrefs would view them with
Pleafure, he giving the Men each a Shilling, and the
Women the fame, to handfel their new Pockets: In
fhort they were publick Beffings, and, indeed, their
Ways were great Delight.

As I was an excellent Horfe-woman, and my Lady
feldom wanted Patients, I arofe two Hours fooner
in the Morning than her Maid ufed to do, and had
my little Pad faddled, fo vifited the Sick every Morning, always telling my Lady what Effects the Medicines had on them that had taken them; this was
great Pleafure to her, for fhe faid that my Judgment
of the Sick exceeded hers. I told her, I was far
from prefuming to vie with her Judgment, but very
defirous of affifting her Patients; and that fhe faid,
fhe was very well affured I would be rewarded here-
after.—So one Morning, as I was upon my Round
vifiting my Sick, behold there came to me a neighbouring bluff Gentleman, having an Eftate of 300 *l.*
per Annum, What, fays he, Miftrefs, are you riding
without

without a Servant to open you the Gates? I need none, Sir, answered I; and there being a Gate just at Hand, I rode up and opened it, so put my Galloway into a Canter: But my Spark being better mounted came up to me, and said, Why so nice, Mistress, I am no Stranger, I have dined many a Time with your Master, and wanted an Opportunity to speak to you: So taking hold on my Bridle, he said, A God it is a Pity you should be a Servant, for you have a Lady's Face, a Face that I could find in my Heart to bestow all my Land on, which is as pretty a Plat of Ground as ever Crow flew over; faith, I have often thought of that Countenance, and am not jesting, said he. And if you was, Sir, I would not take the Advantage of your Jest; go Home and admire your fine Plat of Ground, and don't interrupt me with your Impertinence: So plucked my Bridle out of his Hand, struck into a Gallop and away I went, leaving my Lover with his Plat of fine Land standing like a Scare-crow, and I returned Home another Way. However my Chap came that very Day to dine with my Master, after Dinner he told the Proposals he had made, and the Repartee I gave him; likewise begged of my Master that he would let me know his Designs were honourable, and that he would settle all his Land on me and mine.

My Master promising him his Interest, communicated the whole Story to his Lady, who thought the Proffer very well worth my Acceptance. One Morning she took me into her Closet, and told me what generous Proposals this Gentleman had made my Master, that he would marry me, and settle all his Fortune on me and mine. Madam, answered I, his Proposals I cannot accept, for if his Generosity be great to me, it's slender to his own Posterity; should I bring forth no Children to him, yet have I the Power invested in me to settle all his Fortune on my Relations, and to take that Fortune out of

an

an ancient Family, whofe Chief poffeffed it for fome hundred Years by paft. Well my Dear, faid that good Lady, but in Cafe it fhould be fo, you will have the Power to fettle it on the right Line. But then, Madam, faid I, would not my own Relations have juft Caufe of Complaint, that fuch a Fortune was in my Power as might raife my Family, and I had left it to my Husband's Friends? Befides, I have a more material Objection, and that is, I cannot love the Man were his Fortune ten Times as much as it is; fo I fcorn to accept that Fortune when it is not in my Power to give my Heart in Return. Oh! my dear Girl, anfwered my Miftrefs, thy Sentiments are worthy of Praife, I fhould deprive myfelf of a valuable Servant very willingly, if it had been to thy own Choice; but thou haft a Soul that fcorns an unworthy Thought or Action, only this Fortune might have made thou eafy in Circumftances, and enabled thee to have been helpful to thy fellow Creatures.—But whether fuch a Man would fuffer his Wife fo to do or not, becomes a Query? I fhould be terribly afraid of his bidding me diftribute my own Fortune whenever he beheld my Liberality to the indigent Part of Mankind, and not his amongft Beggars: For which Reafon, if ever I enter into that State, it fhall be with one that I think comes nearer my own Sentiments, and that I am very well affured does not exceed me much in Fortune: I had rather eat the Bread of my Labour and Induftry, than break my Peace for Plenty of Wealth. I efteem Reverence, ferves you honeftly, and is content in my State; would you have me leave a Certainty for an Uncertainty? I might fear the Man but cannot love him, fo will not break my Peace for him. She faid, By no Means, for that was laying a Foundation for a Curfe, and fhe was fure there was a Bleffing in ftore for me. In fhort, my dear Lady told my Mafter my Refolution, he told my Pretender, who took it in fuch Difdain, that he condemned him-

felf

felf for his mean Suit, and faid, He might always have ftoop'd and taken up nothing; that if ever he was flighted again, it fhould be from his Equals, and not an Inferior. My Mafter told me, and I never fee him, and my Miftrefs take fuch a Fit of hearty Laughter. O! Sir, anfwered I, he only ftands condemned as it is, but had he made all his Land over to me and my Heirs, in all likelihood he would have hanged himfelf in fix Months Time. Then, anfwered my Mafter, you would have been a rich young Widow of a large Fortune at your own Difpofal. But I think myfelf ten Times richer as I am, Sir, anfwered I. Then, faid he, in my Opinion your Affections are fixed another Way, which I will leave to your Miftrefs to enquire into, as I don't expect the Difcovery in my hearing; and as he fpoke the Word, walked out of the Room, leaving my worthy Lady with me: Who faid, Is your Mafter right in his Conjecture? I know thy Honour to be frank, and will make no fcruple to make me thy Confident; for if he be more deferving, far be it from me to deprive him of the Happinefs of fo good a Wife, as I am very well affured that thou will be a daily Bleffing to a good Husband.

Thou made me an excellent Cook, and I defire you will inftruct my new Houfe-keeper that it may be kept in the fame Oeconomy; I would not alter the leaft of thy Rule and Order, for I fee very few Tables fet out with that Decorum as mine: Nay, your Mafter has very often told what great Encomiums Gentlemen have given him of my extraordinary Management, whofe Table was fupported with all Rarities in the Seafon, dreffed in the beft Manner, without the leaft Noife or Difturbance; whereas their Houfes were a Hell, their Meat a Surfeit, and the Brauling of Wives and Servants were fo many Tormenters to them. But I have told them all thefe Praifes were due to you, who made all the Houfe

eafy

easy by your Industry and Care, and those who had
such hard Fate as the Torture that such Servants
must give to Masters and Mistresses, I pitied; for if
it was my own Case I should be miserable, the
Integrity and Diligence of Servants, may enable the
Masters to perform the Duty of good and faithful
Stewards. I said, There is certainly great Wisdom
in your Sentiments, Madam; but if every Master
took such Delight in the Duty of the good and
faithful Steward as my Master does, their virtuous
Example would be a great Means to moralize their
Servants: A Manifestation of which is in your own,
you have been nine Years married, and has all your
Servants you first had, but these two that married
from you; every Servant you have is sensible of the
Blessing they daily enjoy, under the Protection of
so virtuous a Master and Mistress. I lived three
Months in three separate Places, quitting the three
Months Wages to be quit of the bad Places, and
have expostulated to my fellow Servants the separate
Tortures that attended those separate Places, which
shew'd them the Difference between good and bad
Places, the Happiness that Servants possessed in the
former, and the Misery of the latter; how well the
Peace and Plenty that we daily enjoy'd deserved our
Diligence and Pains.

Gratitude, the Butler would reply, obliges me to
spur up all my Industry to grace my Master's Table
with clean Plates, Knives, Forks, and Glasses. So
will I, answered the Laundry-maid, with clean Linen.
And, says the Cook, I will feed my Fowls fat, and
will shew my Art of Cookery in dressing the Meat
to grace his Table. And, says I, I will grace it
with a Desert. And says the Dairy-maid, I will
take Care to have good Butter and Cream. The
House-maid replies, My Diligence and Pains shall
be shewn in my clean Rooms, well polished Brasses,
and Irons. Well spoke Fellow-servants, says the
Coachman,

Coachman, my Cattle, Coach, and Harnefs fhall be
as trim. And fo fhall my Saddle Horfes and Furniture, anfwers the Groom. And after all, fays the
Kitchen-maid, I have as much Cleaning as any of you,
and fhall take an equal Share of Pleafure in the Execution of my Duty in the menial Station I enjoy,
under the beft of Mafters, and refpectful fellow Servants. So thou does, anfwered I, and I can obferve a fecret Pleafure to attend you after your Work
is done, as you fit admiring your clean Pots, Pans,
Pewter, Dreffers, &c. &c. fo I am convinced a fecret Pleafure reigns in every Servant's Bofom to difcharge their feveral Duties to thofe two Worthies
they ferve; and who would not think the Prime of
Youth well fpent in the Service of them, that has
the Intereft and well being of their Servants fo much
at Heart? not in the fupporting them with the
Bleffings of this Life, but in fhewing them the Tract
to a better, by their virtuous Example and Goodnefs: For we are not under the Tyranny of cruel
Mafter's horfe-whipping the Men, nor implacable
Miftrefs's tormenting the Maids.

It is very evident, anfwered my Miftrefs, that Servants have as great Souls, and fometimes greater,
than their Mafters. Did not the great and bountiful Giver of all Benefits, according to his wife
Difpenfations to his Creatures, give them their Talents of Wifdom, Riches, Health, Strength, and Underftanding: He did not defign his Bounties of Riches
to be exercifed in Cruelties and Oppreffions, more
efpecially to any Houfhold Servants, whom I efteem
for their Integrity and Care; but you fet them the
Example of Induftry, Gratitude, and Humility, fo
that all the Rule and Order of my Houfe is owing
to your good Prefident; yet, it is my Opinion, I
fhall not have you much longer, by the Anfwer you
made me in the Choice of a Husband, who is to be
near your Fortune and Sentiments: If any Pretender

has

has the Endowments of the latter, it would be a Pity to keep you feparate, although my Lofs will be great that fhall never have fuch a Servant.

You have a compleat Houfewife in your Houfe, a virtuous induftrious Servant, and may confide in her Integrity: I have compleated her as much for the Houfe-keeper as I did the Cook, and her Sifter is as capable to act in the Station of a Cook, fo that you will want only a Kitchen-maid if I leave you: And as I have lived with this honeft Servant near ten Years, can witnefs her Gratitude to Heaven with Tears, for raifing her from fo poor and low a Condition to fo much Peace and Plenty. She has repeated the Extravagancies of her Father, and likewife his Ingratitude to her Mother, who ftole her from her Father's Houfe at Seventeen, which broke his Heart. He died and left a pretty Eftate, which he fpent, and reduced his Wife and Family to the Want of Meat and Cloaths: But the Pains that poor Creature took to relieve thefe unfortunate Diftreffes in her Family, would furprize you. Her eldeft Daughter declares fhe will not run the Risk of her Mother's Hardfhips, for no Man upon Earth, hoping that fhe would difcharge her Duty of Truft in her Place, with that Integrity to her worthy Miftrefs, as fhould not endanger her of lofing it; and likewife to be fo careful of her Wages, as to fave fomething to fupport her after fhe was difabled of performing fervile Duty. If fhe holds faft her Integrity, anfwered my Miftrefs, fhe will be juftly intitled to her Mafter's Bounty, befides mine; who think ourfelves bound in Duty to make Provifion for fuch faithful diligent Servants in their Age, that fpend the Prime of their Youth in our Service: But why did not you inform an of the Diftreffes of her unfortunate Mother? it would have been a Charity done me to have given me Opportunity of relieving her. Madam, anfwered I, fhe told me that her Mother was releafed from
thefe

these Hardships as soon as her Daughters were able to
spin; nor did she ever let her Wants be known, even
in the greatest Distress, after her Father obliged
her to sign the Right of all her Fortune to him.
He sold it, and went over to *France*, and never returned again, leaving her with four Daughters, the Eldest
of them being but five Years of Age. But this industrious Mother has not let her Daughters spend
their Time in Indolence nor Vanity, you have two
of them, which, in my Opinion, are as good Servants as any in *England*. That is owing to you their
Teacher, for their Mother might teach them Spin-
ning, Knitting, and Sowing, but her low Station of
Life disabled her from compleating them of Cookery
and Housewifery : That valuable Treasure you
possess beyond most of Women in Oeconomy and
compleat Housewifery, which you have so frankly
bestowed on these Girls, must lay them and me under great Obligations to you : For there are very
few so generous of their Knowledge in the Art of
Cookery, as to give *gratis* what others would not
part with for Money : Heaven was kind in bestow-
ing such a Servant on me, that has intailed Decorum
and good Order in my Family. I answered, 'Twas
a double Duty incumbent on me, in Gratitude to
the best of Mistresses, so humane, charitable, and
benevolent, whose good Works I daily admired,
and would imitate to the best of my Ability. My
Mother gave 20 *l.* and three Years Service to a
Pastry Cook with me, at the 15th Year of my Age:
I am now 30, and have improved my Talent. In this
Servant I beheld a generous Soul full of Industry and
Gratitude, and took great Pleasure in communicating
to her my Instructions and Advice; she has been so
quick of Apprehension, that she improved what I
taught her, has instructed her Sister, and you'll find
her exceed me; having now in her Possession all I
could teach her, besides a fruitful Head of her own.

So

So my dear Lady told me, If I had had her Fortune, how far I would have exceeded her in good Works; and said, She rejoiced she had such good and worthy Servants, trained up by my Instructions. And now, said she, as all your Sentiments are frank, let me know what happy Man engages your Affections, and how long he has possessed that Treasure: You need not blush, for I am convinced he is a virtuous Lover. I answered, That I had great Reason to believe him such, he is a Mechanick, Madam, says I: His Master was that Architecture that undertook all the Building of this House, Out-offices, School-house, &c. he was Foreman over the Work, and employed three Years in this Building, being boarded in the Steward's House, a Relation of his: And when his first Son was made a Christian, I was desired to stand Godmother, and this Youth was a Godfather.

Although he had a beautiful Person and Behaviour, yet I did not much mind him, nor even knew him, although he had wrought near three Years in the Building, and had my Orders for making the Conveniencies of the Store-room, Laundry, and Dairy: He having a quick Genius, and diligently observed my Directions, yet I never gave him the Applause that I generally gave the other Artists, left he might have some secret Vanity of thinking that he merited my Esteem; which was so far from it, that I did not know him to be the Man, till the Steward asked him how long the Work would be in finishing. He answering, In a Month's Time, and that will make out three Years the Workmen have been employed in the Improvements your worthy Master has made about his House. So, said I, is this the young Man that made all my Conveniencies in my Store-room and other Places: Indeed, I beg Pardon, for I have not seen you since you finished my Apartment, so that I had quite forgot you.
But

But, said he, I wish you had been no more significant in my Esteem, than I have been in yours, and perhaps I might have forgot you also. Sir, answered I, It is not worth the Notice of your Sex, let my Significancy be less or more, they are not to be better or worse for it.

Early the next Morning I received a Letter from him, the Contents of which set forth the Beauty of his Wisdom, and likewise the Purity of his Affection, which, in serious Words, declared that he was a Stranger to Love before, but has been captivated ever since he first beheld me. I was diverted with reading the Beginning of his Letter, but surprized at the Conclusion of it; for upon Reflection, I found he had a Store of Judgment and Understanding, and could not help condemning myself for my rude haughty Behaviour to him, still, in spite of all my Resolutions, admiring the Dictates of his Brain: It was a Week before I could have Time to send him an Answer, which was to the following Effect.

SIR,

" The Perusal of Yours gave me an Opportunity of seeing how erroneous I was in my Conjectures, for having never seen so great a Number of House-carpenters and Joiners working in one House, as we had when that Wing was built to my Master's, where a Gallery Window gave me an Opportunity of seeing the Workmen act at their separate Branches, hammering, sawing, glewing, plaining, and some singing, whistling, others cursing and swearing; the Noise of whose Pipes and Voices rendered me in *Bedlam.* Indeed sometimes I could scarce think them rational, for as one young Man was rapping upon his Plain with a Hammer, while he was whistling a Tune, and raising his Note so high as I thought the Extent of the Pipe, affected his Sight for rapping upon the Piece of Wood that he had been rubbing upon

the

the Deal, out flies a Piece of Iron and pitched upon his Ancle, which cut him to the Bone. I sent
for him immediately, and washed it with some Balsam, and bid him whistle after his Work-hours were
over, as he was not able to whistle, work, and think,
to any Perfection at once: Nor did I think you, their
deputed Master, had your Men in such Decorum as
they ought to have been in your Presence, as Ham-
mers, Axes, Adges, &c. makes Noise enough without whistling, singing, cursing, and swearing; so that
I looked on your Fraternity to be a robust Sort of
uncoth People, till after the Perusal of your Letter,
in which I perceive you are Master of a good Stock
of Reasoning, and, as far as my Judgment goes, seems
to tell a Story of Love very well, although I think
it's a dangerous Suit for a handy-craft Tradesman to
make with a House-keeper of such a Family, as I
have the Honour of serving, where every Servant is
as happy as they wish to be, by the Indulgence of
the best and humblest of Masters. This may make
proud Servants, or at least you may think so, by the
Resolution that I have taken, which is this, that I
never will marry a Man before he has maintained a
seven Years Conversation in Letters, during which
Time, he shall not importune me with one personal
Visit. Once a Month I will receive a Letter, and
no oftner; every tenth Letter I will answer, and no
more; nor will I give him any Assurance of Marriage at the seven Years End. Now my Heart is
free, nor was it ever entangled; nor do I design to
yield it to any Man, that dares to intrude, or make
the least Breach of any Article that I propose unto
him. So, Sir, as your Business will be finished in
three Weeks, I will receive a Letter from your Messenger at your Departure, and not before."

Now, Madam, the seven Years is within the
last Month of the Expiration, without the Breach
of Covenant on either Side, and if I was an Empress
Queen,

Queen, he fhould be my Sovereign. I beg you will give me the Perufal of his fecond and laft Letters, faid my dear Miftrefs, which I did: Now, faid fhe, while I am reading thefe Letters, do you let the Servants know what different Stations they are to ferve me in. So communicating the Whole to the Cook, fhe acknowledged with Tears the Benefits that fhe had received from me. I told her that it did not impoverifh me, what Benefits fhe had got by me gave the utmoft Pleafure to my Soul, to make her fit to ferve that dear Angel of a Woman: As alfo, that it was in my Power to do you that Service, which if I had not when Time was, could not do it now, my Time being expired. Well, anfwered fhe, you muft receive the Reward of good Works, that never omitted any Opportunity of doing that Duty; and I hope you will receive the Reward of your good Works, in that State you are near entering into. As your Goodnefs has been fo great to us, I hope you will add to thefe Obligations already received, aud that is accepting of a third Sifter for a Servant; you will find fhe has Integrity, and a Genius that you will have Pleafure of improving; was rather the Favourite of my Mother, for her fuperior Care and Induftry: She was the Market-maker, and fhe will fhew you the Way to be rich by Frugality.

That is fuch a Servant as I fhall want very much, for I know not how to act in the low Station of Life, after living fo long amongft great Plenty: Very few Noblemen live better, fome not near the Plenty of this Family. She will fhew Thrift—Juft as fhe fpoke, my Miftrefs's Bell rung, up I went, and fhe fmiling faid, I am afraid I will become troublefome to you for Favours. I wifh'd it were in my Power to oblige, anfwered I, Madam command me. Then, faid fhe, let me have the fame Liberty of all your Love Letters, that I have had of thefe two, and your Mafter to read them. If you defire it, I
faid.

faid. I do, my good Girl, anfwered fhe, fo I gave her them with all the Copies of mine, which they read with Attention. So when I dreffed my Miftrefs next Day, fhe very complaifantly returned me my Letters, and told me how much they were furprized with the Courtfhip: Declaring that you have great Senfe, and the Art of Reafoning, that exceeds moft of Women; yet he thinks you have put your Lover under fuch Reftrictions as is amazing, and folemnly declares, that you fhall fall very low in his Efteem, if you keep him any longer in Sufpence. In fhort, added fhe, it furprized me how you found out fuch Objections, or could withftand the Pleadings of this Man. Who, your Mafter fays, may plead a Caufe with a Lawyer at the Bar: Such is his Wit and Reafoning, as drew Tears from both our Eyes. He knows the young Man, his Mafter is a Man generally efteemed for his Integrity and Behaviour, and you know very well, he never came here but your Mafter paid him as much Refpect as any Gentleman that came to his Houfe; he is acknowledged to be the greateft Architect in this Country, and he lives ten Miles from us.

There is a Farm of your Mafter's, that his Predeceffors obliged their Heirs, not to let that Farm to any other Tenant, than he that lived on it at that Time, who was a Servant that married from the Family; nor had the Heirs Power to raife the Rent: This Tenant is a very old Man, and the laft of the Family, that has enjoyed this Farm two Hundred Years. He has taken a Ride out this Morning, and bid me not wait Dinner for him; fo, I fuppofe, he is gone to pay his old Tenant a Vifit, and very likely may give your fuppofed Mafter a Call. This is Conjecture, but if it fhould happen to prove Truth, and he bring Home your Lover, how would you receive him?

Nay,

Nay, Madam, anſwered I, if he has ſo worthy an Introductor, he needs not fear a hearty Welcome: But I cannot have the Vanity to think myſelf deſerving ſuch Notice. You deſerve the Reſpect, due to ſo good and faithful a Servant, an Example of virtuous Induſtry. I ſurprized your Maſter with the Account I gave him of your Management of the Feathers, and what Pleaſure it gave me to ſee your Particulars in the Order and Care of picking them off every Fowl: All the Pens you kept ſeparate from ſmall Feathers; the Geeſe and Ducks you put together; Turkeys, Hens, and Chickens you mix them together, and after your Fowls were bled, tied up the Wound with a coarſe Rubber, left any of the Blood dropt amongſt the Feathers: Had ſeparate Bags to put them in, as ſoon as they were plotted, which Bags were hung upon Hooks in the Ceiling of the Kitchen; and after Houſhold Bread had been baked in the Oven, and the Oven of a moderate Warmth, you put in theſe Bags to dry the Feathers thoroughly, as alſo to deſtroy any Thing quick, amongſt ſuch Feathers. That you had fitted me ſix Beds of Gooſe and Duck Feathers, not inferior to live Feathers; and that you had as many of Turkey, Hen, Capon, and Chicken Feathers as would fill four Beds more, not ſo good as the Duck and Gooſe Feathers; but by the Care and good Management of them, in drying them in the Oven, and thereby not only ſeaſoning, but deſtroying ſuch Vermin as feathered Fowls are ſubject to, and keeping the Pens and great Feathers from each other, they would make four very good Beds.

And, my Dear, anſwered he, ſhe very well deſerves them with Furniture to them, viz. Quilts, Ticks, Blankets, &c. For, my Dear, added he, Induſtry is an Emblem of Virtue, that merits Reward. So accordingly I have ordered the above-named to
the

the Upholfterer; and as your Feathers need no dreffing, having taken Care of that before-hand, by
your skilful Management, they are ready to put into the Ticks, and I will fit you out four Beds. As
you took Care to employ the poor People in fpin-
ning, fo I have a Stock of Webs by me, and I intend you four for Sheets; you know their Lengths,
forty-four Yards each, two of fine, and two of
coarfe: So fhall you have alfo a Web of Diaper, and
one of Hugaback for Table-cloths; befide fome
other Neceffaries, that I fhall think on after. Dear
Madam, faid I, how is it poffible for me to receive
fuch Bounties? I am not covetous, nor can be eafy
to become fo great a Charge upon you: The Perquifites of your Place fupplied me with Neceffaries;
and I have my ten Years Wages untouched, which
will do more than furnifh my Houfe; and have gathered enough under the Shadow of your Generofity, to anfwer fundry Purpofes, and in a conjugated
State, why would you load me with more? Your
Goodnefs and Generofity is great in beftowing, and
I am abafhed as a Receiver; certainly my Husband
and I, if we draw equally in the Yoke, may acquire
Bread.

I therefore know the Franknefs of thy Soul, faid
fhe, for obferving the Maids all very neat at the
Chapel, I perceived them all dreffed in the Gowns,
Handkerchiefs, Aprons, Ruffles, and Head Suits I
had given you, and asking the Chamber-maid, what
fhe paid you for the Gown and Linen that you had
on laft *Sunday?* Nothing at all, anfwered fhe, Madam
the Houfe-keeper faid you lent them to her to give
to us: But whatever fhe gives us of yours, fhe bids
us look on as facred; nor do we wear any Thing
that was yours, in any other Place but the Church,
and as foon as Divine Service is over, we all undrefs
ourfelves, and put on our Homefpun Gowns, fo folds
up our Clothes, which fhe very diligently obferves;
for

for no Maid in the Family she allows above one
Gown washed in a Quarter of a Year: So every
one of us endeavours which shall keep their Gown
cleanest. All this I told your Master, which pleased
him so well, that the first Chapman that came with
a Horse-pack, he bought me three Webs of the best
Chintz Gottons; and said, Make Plenty of these
Gowns, wear them a while in the Mornings, and
cast them to your Maid, who very well deserves
to have the Distribution of them. But this Injunction I lay you under, that you shall not distribute
any of my Castings, that I give you at this Juncture;
for altho' you have a great Soul, your intended Husband has not your Master's Fortune to support it:
But go and order Dinner to be ready at Two o'Clock,
your Master was on Horseback at Six, and we will
stay Dinner one Hour, in Expectation of his coming. This stunn'd me a little; but was more surprized at the Approach of my Master and Lover entering into the Court: The Steward seeing them,
said, Behold, I will wager something there is a Building on the Anvil; for here is my Gossip Cousin,
and I hear my Master cry aloud for Dinner. The
Cook answers it is very ready for him, although it
be half an Hour before my Orders for it: Although
no Soul in the House had the least Knowledge of
the Story, yet my Confusion was such, as I believed
them all privy to the whole Affair; so stepping into the Store-room, in order to hide it, and set
up the cold Things for the Table, in comes the Butler for them, and says, Mistress, this is the Youth
that was Foreman over the Carpenters and Joiners,
in these Buildings of ours; I think him a pretty
young Man, and the genteelest Mechanick that e-
ver I see: I can tell you that there are some Esquires
that visits my Master's that has not his Deportment,
nor seeming Candour; every Word he speaks has
Grace and Sweetness in it; he eats nothing; Master
obliged him to drink two Glasses of Wine, and Ma-

ster

ster and Lady seems to take Abundance of Notice
of him. Perhaps, said I, they want to set forward
some Building. Very likely, said he, and took in
the Desert.

As soon as we Servants were set down to Dinner,
Orders came from my Mistress, that she wanted me
after I had dined : Accordingly I did, being then quite
serene, I entered the Drawing-room ; yet all my
Resolution of Serenity departed at the first Glimpse
of my Lover, I was in such a Confusion when he
made a low Bow to me, such a Heat struck into
my Face, as I never found in the greatest Dinner I
ever drest. My Master, smiling said, Behold there
is Virtue in the highest Perfection : So taking me
by the Hand, bid me sit down, having something
of Moment to communicate to me. Sir, answered I,
I am unacquainted with sitting in your Presence.
But you must sit now, said my Master. I giving
a wishful Look to my Mistress, who said, Oblige
me in obeying your Master ; and with a reverend
Kneel I did sit down. Now, says he, before your
Story comes upon the Carpet, I have something to
say to your Mistress : Thus he began, I think, my
Dear, I told you, that I would take a Ride to see
my old Tenant that People have been importuning
me a long Time to take the Farm at the Expiration
of his Lease : I went to see this old Tenant, and
found him sitting in an easy Chair, propt with Pil-
lows, and all Things very clean and neat about him ;
seeing me the old Woman seem'd pleased, and bid
a Woman, that had been his Servant, take a Key,
open a Cupboard-door, and bring him a Paper that
was lying on the Bottom of this little Cupboard,
which she accordingly did : He taking it in his
Hand, said, Sir, my Predecessors have enjoyed this
Farm without Molestation these two Hundred Years ;
although the Farm was worth more Rent than we
paid, the Rent was not raised : I being the last of
the

the Family, that hath acquired a Fortune of four Thousand Pounds, I mean, said he, what my Father left me at his Death, and what I have by Care and Industry added to it, and I was bound in Conscience, Gratitude, and Duty to the Family, from whence this Fortune was raised, (having no Tie of Blood to share any of my Effects) have made you my Executor. So gave me his last Will, and delivered the Key of his Securities: He seemed pleased when he took his last Leave of me, and said, Sir, I hope we'll meet again in Heaven; where if your Forefathers have not Mansions of Glory, what must become of me? Tears trickling down the old Man's Cheeks, which forced Tears from my Eyes, to see the Dissolution of an upright honest Man approach; who said, That he wished that the Minister would come, it was near the Time, that I might join in a Petition to Heaven for him. Accordingly I did, and with a humble Voice joined the venerable old Man, who exalted his, as if the Soul had been upon its Flight to it's Place of Rest. When Prayers were done, with Tranquillity of Mind he thanked the Minister, that had taken great Care of discharging the Duty of the Physician of the Soul; which I hope by your pious Instructions, and my own Endeavours make my Soul fit for it's Change, which will, in my Opinion, be in a short Time: I finding myself very weak, hopes not to give you much more Trouble, as I find my Strength failing very fast: I have, Sir, turning his Eyes to me, left that good Man a Legacy in my Will, he having but a very small Living, and five Children; if you think it too small you have it in your Power to add to it: So saying, beckened as tho' he wanted to be at Rest.

The Priest and I departed, he lamenting the Loss that he would sustain onto worthy and honest a Neighbor. Then [ ] I. He is going to receive the reward of his good Works. [ ] an-

{wered the Prieft, has lived to a great Age ; but I am afraid that I ftand a very great Hazard of lofing as worthy a Man, that hath not lived half the Number of his Years: I think they will not leave fuch two behind them in my whole Parifh. I asked him who this Gentleman was. He anfwered, That he was the greateft Architecture in the Country, and naming him. I faid, That I had a Number of his Men employed in building for me: The Death of fo worthy a Man will be a general Lofs ; is there any immediate Danger? I can perceive him alter, turns pale, and is not able to give that due Atttendance to the Church, as he always was accuftomed to, when in Health. What is his Complaint, Sir? faid I. He anfwered, That the Doctor was afraid of a Confumption, occafioned by the Death of his Wife, that he loved, and they lived in fuch Happinefs, that all his Refolutions could not fupport him under his immoderate Grief: So that it is thought he is labouring under the Anguifh of a broken Heart. How far are we from his Houfe? faid I. He anfwered, Two Miles. Will you fhew me the Way to his Houfe? Sir, faid he, it is near to a fick Perfon that I have to adminifter the Sacrament to. So when we came to the Place, the Prieft fhewed me the Houfe, that this worthy Man lived at ; which was on the direct Road: He would have rid with me, but I bid him vifit his Sick, and I would be glad to fee him after, as I could not go wrong.

Leaving the Prieft, I rid up to the Houfe, rapp'd at the Door, and out comes the Maid: I asked her if her Mafter was at Home. She faid, He was, but not very well. Is he up? faid I. She anfwered, He was: But he feeing me come to the Door, I was amazed to fee fuch a Change as there was in him ; for if I had feen him from Home, I fhould not have known him: But notwithftanding his Illnefs, he feemed rejoiced to fee me ; and begged that

I

I would go in, which I very willingly did; telling him, That I was very forry to fee him indifpofed, but hoped he would get the better of it, as I partly was informed of the Reafon, which might go off in Time. He faid, He feared it would not, as he found himfelf weaken every Day. Sir, faid I to him, you muft not die; in fhort we cannot want you: Therefore get well, and build me another Wing to my Houfe. Sir, anfwered he, I have inftructed a Youth in all the different Rules and Branches of Architecture, whofe Integrity and Judgment you may confide in: He was left to me an Orphan, by his dying Father, who begged of me to adopt him my Son; he having no other Parent, and all he had to leave him was one Hundred Pounds, which he had good Security for.

He was feven Years of Age when I took him from his Father, and did adopt him my Son; nor have I drawn any Intereft of his Hundred Pounds, and he is now thirty Years of Age, and has one Hundred Pounds of his own Wages out at Intereft: But what is this Trifle of Money, to his intrinfick Worth? which has been the Key of my Truft, ever fince he got his Education, and entered into his Apprenticefhip: No Son could be more dutiful to a Father, nor did I love any of my three Sons better than him, and he has a noble Mind. But, Sir, I have obferved him more thoughtful for thefe two Months paft than ufual, and taking him into my Clofet, afked what it was that fretted him, and told him, That I heard as a very great Secret, that he fent Letters by a fpecial Meffenger to your Houfekeeper, and that I thought he would not conceal any Thing from me; adding, that it would add to my Sorrow, if I fhould look little in his Eyes. He fell down on his Knees, and faid, I call Heaven to witnefs if filial Affections ever diminifhed; all your Afflictions were Oppreffion to my Soul: I have petitioned

titioned Heaven to take that Load of Sorrow from you, and lay on me, and yet this dear Creature you mention, hath rivalled you about ten Years in my Love. I answered, My dear Son, I very willingly submit to my Rival, and nothing would be a greater Temptation for me to wish for Life more, than to see thee married to so virtuous, worthy and industrious a Woman as she is. I have so little Hope, answered he, that I altogether despair of ever being so happy. I asked him when he saw her. His Answer was, Not these seven Years. Says I, How should you hope to get her, if you have not been in her Company for seven Years. That was not my Fault, said he, for I would have tramp'd through Frost and Snow on my bare Feet, to be one Hour in her Company, with her own Consent: But such was the Restraint she laid me under, and if I made the least Breach of any one Article, it should be a total Discharge. Her Commands were these, that she would marry no Man, that did not solicit her seven Years in Writing; nor would she receive any more Letters from him but one every Month, and that she would give Answer to every tenth Letter, and no oftner; her last Letter seems full as indifferent as the first. Let me read it, said I.

He brought me it, and indeed, Sir, I never saw a Letter wrote by a Woman that contained so much Judgment and good Sense: I bid him not despair, for as she possessed a great Share of Reason, so good a Creature cannot be void of Love and Honour, that will reward all thy Pains. He told me it would not be his Fortune to get such a Woman; otherwise she could not have tortured so long a Time what she loved.

Let me see this despairing Man, answered I: He came just in his working Clothes. I said, Young Man, you may put on another Coat, and ride Home with

with me, I have to treat with you in a building Affair. He made a very low Bow, and faid he would be ready in a Minute. Scarce had his Mafter and I drunk a Difh of Coffee till we faw the Horfe ftanding at the Door; his Mafter whifpered me not to let him know the Contents of our Converfation; nor did I difcover the leaft Word till this Inftant. Now, as the greateft Prudence has conducted every other Action of yours, we can witnefs, fince you came into this Family; nor do I at all difpute but that you have a fecret Reafon for this terrible Courtfhip, that you have contrived: And as there is a Franknefs in you, give us the Motive that induced you to it; for had your Miftrefs put me under fuch feven Years Penance, fhe had fet me diftracted.

I with great Compofure anfwered, Circumftances altered Cafes; yours, Sir, and that good Lady were the Off-fpring of two worthy Families, had both the Benefit of liberal Educations and bountiful Fortunes, have two Bodies and one Mind, poffeffed with every Blefling under Heaven, whofe Light fo fhines, that we, your Servants, that daily behold your good Works with Praife and Admiration, would very ill deferve thefe Benefits, if we quit them for Uncertainties: As I was intrufted with the Diftribution of fome Part of your Charity, to the Relief of the diftreffed, which gave me the Profpect of the different Characters of the loweft Clafs of Mankind. In vifiting the Sick, for which my Miftrefs gave me two Hours every Day, I found more Diftempers proceed from churlifh Husbands, than any other Caufe; fome in drinking, when their Wives and Children are ftarving for Meat and Clothes. Carrying fome Relief to a poor Widow, with four Children lying in the Small-pox, who begged of me to call at a Cottage, a Quarter of a Mile from her Houfe, There, fays fhe, is a pretty young Creature in great Diftrefs, who was deluded from her Mother's

Houfe

House by a young wild Fellow, a Carpenter; who got her perſwaded to marry him, under ſpecious Pretences of keeping her like a Lady, and as ſoon as ſhe was in his full Power, and abandoned by all her Friends, put her into that poor Cottage, without Furniture, except two Stools, a Bedſtead, and Bed without Curtains. He came Home laſt Night, and brought her a Leg of Mutton, which ſhe boiled to his Dinner: She having a Neighbour, Wife to a prodigal Bricklayer, who had left her with a Child ſucking on her Breaſt, without Meat, or Money; ſhe begged Leave of her Husband, to let her give the poor Woman a Morſel of Meat and a Meſs of Broth; which he enraged with Fury, ſwore he had a Charge great enough of maintaining her, and do you bring more upon me, the feeding your Neighbours; and furiouſly ſtruck her on the Head, and cut her with a Knife to the Skull. I knowing of the Diſtreſs of the Bricklayer's Wife, who is a Relation to me, carried her a Pint of Milk and a Barley-cake, which ſhe could not eat, although dying of Hunger. I hearing the bitter Cries of the Woman, went into the Houſe, and found her in the greateſt Agony of Grief, all beſmeared with Blood, ſhe telling me the Words that I have already repeated to you.

This being *Sunday* Evening, I had taken the Groom to ride before me, I thought it lucky to have a Man with me on ſuch an Errand, ſo rode up to this Cottage: I lighted from my Horſe, went into the Houſe, and to my great Surprize found this pretty young Creature to be a Tenant's only Daughter of yours; ſhe ſeeing me, diſcharged a freſh Flood of Tears, and ſaid, Oh! that I had died, rather than I ſhould have given the Pain of my Hardſhips to a Heart ſo humane as yours. But let me eaſe that Pain, by dreſſing your Wound; you need not tell me how you got it, I know who gave it you, and
for

for what. So cutting away the Hair, washed the
Wound with a little warm Water, to take the Blood
from it, making it clean, laid some Balsam to it, and
put a Bandage round her Head. Now, said I, you
are eased of the Pain, let me know how you came
by this Bargain. In a great Hurry, said she, For
you must know my Mother was so much afraid of
me, that she would not trust me out of her Sight,
hired a Woman to teach reading, writing, and sew-
ing, and so brought about this Bargain; after she
had taught me all she was able, then she recommended this Man, as one whose Father had a great Estate,
and that he might keep me as grand as any Lady: I
was easily prevailed on to make this run away Wedding; she thought to persuade my Mother to take
me Home, but has found herself mistaken, for instead of giving her any further Credit, made all Enquiry after her Character, and has found her to be
an Impostor, and a common Prostitude, that had
born this Man to another poor Woman's Husband,
when she was but twenty Years of Age; was a kept
Mistress, very grand by a Gentleman, till his Death;
but he leaving her no Subsistance, she was abandoned
by all that knew her; yet having a Relation that
was an Intimate of my Mother's, which she came
to in great Distress. This Woman recommended her
as a virtuous understanding Woman, very fit to instruct me, as she was Mistress of her Needle; and
such was the Credulity of my Mother, that she took
her into her House, gave her three Pounds a Year,
and kept her seven Years teaching me. She for her
own private Views got me matched to her Son, that
is not so quick sighted as his Mother, vulgarly wicked, and tyranically cruel: He was beating me one
Day, when one of his Companions came in, and
asked him what Crime I had committed. He answered, None: I give her this Exercise for my own
Diversion, and to make her an obedient Wife; a
Woman, a Dog, and an Ive Tree, beat them well,
and

and the better they will be. Curfe on all Wives!
a Curfe on my Mother, that bound me to one! Was
not thou and I far better fingle? We were far better, anfwered the other; come go Home with me,
and I will beat my Wife to make her good: Thee
and me will get ourfelves drunk, and let them weep on.

I faid, Can you love this Man after all this ty-
ranizing he treats you with? Love him! anfwered
fhe, no, but dreads him as much as a Serpent. But
had you not better make an Elopement from him,
and go to your Mother, that muft love you. But
how can I have the Affurance to look my Mother
in the Face, after I have given her fo much Dif-
grace and Sorrow by my Ingratitude. I anfwered,
If I fhould procure your Mother's Pardon, and
fhe be willing to receive you into her former Favour,
and take you from this Husband that ufes you
fo ill, could you be content to live without him?
Yes, and fit down on my Knees, and pray for my
Deliverance from a Brute; would know better how
to value my Bleffings, and pay my Duty to the beft
of Mothers, that has lived a Widow fixteen Years,
although fhe might have been married to very refpon-
fable Men, which fhe refufed; told them that they
would not court a Widow, but on Expectation of
a lumping Bargain; that they fhould not impair my
Fortune one Farthing, and that fhe never would
give any Man her Hand, as fhe had no Heart to
give. I therefore do pay that Honour due to her
with a penitent Heart. But pray tell me, anfwered
I, what Situation of Life is your Neighbour in. She
is Wife to that Companion of my Husband's, faid
fhe, and the more miferable in one Refpect, for
having a Child fucking on her Breaft, fhe requires
more Food than his fmall Matter which he gives
her will procure, it being but one Shilling a Week,
although he can earn nine Shillings *per* Week. Have
you no better Salary. No; but I have a Joint of
fome

some Sort of Butcher's Meat, which I always boil, and makes Broth, to help my Neighbour with; whose Husband perhaps will not see her for a Month, as he sends her Salary with my Bargain: One Time I complained of the small Matter for a Wife and a Child, and he damn'd both her and me, bidding us work for more.

These three Days past we had but a Penny Loaf, and three Pints of Milk betwixt us, and if you were sensible of the Pain that poor Mortal complains of when she wants Food, the Child crying for the Breast, to still it's Complaint, gives it the empty Breast to suck: And she says, the Child pulling and drawing her Breast when there is no Milk in it, is just tearing her Heart out, and raises such Cholicks, and Wind at her Stomach, as renders her miserable. Vexation and Hunger I think seems to get the better of her Constitution, for if after a long Fast she eats, it seems to give her Pain instead of Refreshment; and what frets me more is, that I shall share the same Fate, as I am seven Months gone with Child. You hope for Relief, answered I, and direct me to your distressed Neighbour, if you can point me out the Entrance, as you are not able to go with me. I think you have given me new Spirits, answered she, to shew you the Door; we live both under one Roof, yet the Doors open contrary, the one in the Backside of the House, and the other in the Foreside. Entering the House, beheld it more decently furnished, yet a more melancholy Prospect, for the Mother and Child were perfect Skeletons; the feeble Mother had boiled the Pint of Milk with the Bread, the poor Widow had carried her, and the poor meagre Infant ravenously fought for it's Food, when the feeble Mother was not able to feed it; nor had she Spirits to speak to me. I saw the Tears in her Eyes, but hearing her

Story

Story before, I did not diſturb her with asking
Queſtions.

I bid them both hope for better, Providence was
a wonderful Supporter of all thoſe who put their
Truſt in him : So taking my Leave of them, rode
Home in all Haſte, and ſent a poor Woman, that
was employed in weeding the Gardens, with two
Bottles of Malt Liquor, a Loaf of Bread, ſome Sugar, gave her Money to buy Milk and Butter, and
directed her to this Cottage; bid her make Poſſets
of the Malt Liquor, Bread, Sugar, and Milk, then
give the Woman Bread and Butter, ſtay by her and
keep the Child, and take the ſame Care you do of
other ſick People till I ſee you.

Then, Madam, I came to you, and told you that
one of your Tenants had been under a lingering Ill-
neſs for ſome Time, and deſired Leave to viſit her :
You asked which of your Tenants; I anſwered the
prudent Widow, that brought her beautiful Daughter to ſee you. By all Means go, if it be not too late,
for 'tis twelve Miles. I have Time enough, Madam, anſwered I. So I was ordered to take ſome
Cordials, very proper for many Complaints; away
I went on a very good double Horſe, which was
made ready : Having a good Guide we got there
before they were in Beds, and although the honeſt
Woman was labouring under the greateſt Affliction,
yet ſhe forgot it at the Sight of me ; who ſhe got
in her Arms, and ſaid, What good Star has conducted thee to my Habitation? I anſwered, If you
will order my Guide cold Meat, me a Morſel of
Bread and Butter, and retire with me into your
Lodging-room, you ſhall have the Contents of my
Progreſs. She ſpreading a Cloth on the Table,
ordered her Maid to bring on the cold Beef, Bacon, and Veal and a large Diſhful ſhe brought her
Miſtreſs; telling me at the ſame Time, that this
was

was the general Custom of the Farmers, to boil as much Meat one Day, as would serve them three Dinners: For, added she, our Time is taken up in taking Care of our Cattle and Corn, we spend very little Time in Cooking.

So taking me by the Hand, led me into a very neat Parlour, with a clean Fire-side; set out a little Table, laid a Cloth, and brought a cold Pigeon Pye, a large Short-cake, a very good Cheese, a Bottle of red *Port*, and a Bottle of white Wine, and said, Blessed be that Landlord, that lets his Tenants such Farms, as will enable them to give their Friend such a hearty Welcome: For I can tell you, very few Tenants enjoy the Blessings of Plenty that your Master's Tenants do, my Servants live better than many Masters, that farms in this Country; I would very ill deserve the Blessing of such a Landlord, not to acknowledge it. Here is one Esquire *Stony-heart*, that lives in this Neighbourhood, the Plantation Slaves are more happy than his Tenants: One of them came to me last Week, brought with him a twenty Years Lease of his Farm, three Years of which being expired, and told me, That he having been at a great Expence in improving his Farm, which appeared in this Year's Crop; behold, one of his Landlord's Vassals kept by him as a Spy came, and seeing us very busy sheering; told me, That I had forgot my Rent-day. I answered, That they certainly never broke the Term that came on the Morrow. All the Damage would only be paying up the whole Year's Rent, or forfeit the Lease, answered he.

Upon this the poor Man came in the greatest Confusion, brought with him the half Year's Rent, due the Day before, which his last Receipt testified; and begging of me to read his Lease to him, which I did: Upon Perusal I found that he entered this

Farm

Farm the firſt Day of *May*, the yearly Rent 80 *l.*
which firſt half Year's Rent was to be paid on *Can-
dlemas-day*, and the other on *Lammas-day*; the Non-
payment of the Rent on theſe two individual Days,
for ſuch Default the Landlord ſhould be entitled to
have his full Year's Rent paid by the Tenant on Demand, or have his Goods and Chattels ſeized upon the
Premiſes; that ſuch Goods and Chattels ſhould be
praized and ſold the next Day to the beſt Bidder:
And if theſe Goods and Chattels did not amount to
a full Year's Rent, the Leaſe to be void, and of no
Effect. I thought the honeſt induſtrious Man would
have dropp'd down: Fear not, Man, ſaid I, I will
lend thee as much Money as thy half Year's Rent,
and go pay him up, and bid Eſquire *Stony-heart* Defiance: He wants to reap the Profit of thy Improvements; which, as one of thy Neighbours told me,
had coſt thee 150 *l*. As I ſpoke the Word, came a
Son of this Farmer, and told his Father that the Fellow that was ſpeaking to him, with two more in
Company, were driving all the Cattle out of the
Paſture, and no doubt, ſaid the Boy, will ſell *Robin
Hood*'s Pennyworths To-morrow, beſides the trick-
ing you out of your Leaſe. No, Son, I bid them
Defiance, and thanks God for a worthy Friend, that
will reſcue me.

So I lent him the Money, and bid him tell Eſquire
Stony-heart, that he had not a Tenant that was able
to do ſuch an Act of Humanity, as a Tenant of E-
ſquire *Goodman*'s did, who lent thee 40 *l*. to pray
for long Life to her Landlord, and that rejoiced to
ſee his Tenants live; and to pray for Reformation
to all the Family of *Stony-heart*'s, that are Oppreſſors
of their Tenants, as he is.

The Man went to pay his ignoble Landlord, full
of Joy, and I was as well pleaſed to have the Opportunity of doing an honeſt Man ſuch a Service:

I

I don't speak this out of Oftentation; for when I enquired into the State of my Soul, I found but very little Provifion made for it; for this Daughter that my Vanity prompted me to fhew in a Vifit to the worthy Family of yours, thinking to charm your dear Lady with her Beauty as much as fhe did me. I made her the Idol of my Soul, was deaf to any Complaints of Diftreffes, left the relieving them fhould impair this Daughter's Subftance. I told thofe in Diftrefs, who defired my Help, That I was only a Stewardefs to my Daughter, and would not run the Risk of impairing the Bounty of Fortune which Providence had intrufted me with, I would not let any Mortal converfe with her.

In all Sorts of Needle-work, Reading, Writing, Mufiek, both *German* Flute, and Violin, Dancing, *&c.* I had her inftructed by a Woman, recommended to me by a Relation of her's, and a pretended Friend of mine: Thus through too great an Excefs of Credulity I became impofed on, admitting only fhe, my Daughter's Affociate. When my Daughter was dreffed, and danced a Minuet, I was fo much charmed with her, that I was afraid to let her be feen, left every one that beheld her, fhould covet robbing me of her. If I took her to Church, I muffled her Face up fo clofe, that none could tell what Sort of a Face fhe had, and fet her in a Pew that I bought for the concealing her from the Sight of the Congregation; it ftood one Half facing the Minifter and People, the other Part ftanding behind them in that Part where fhe fits. I told her that when fhe went into the Houfe of God, it was to pray, and not to gaze, or be gazed at by the Congregation.

When her Father died, he left us worth 600 *l.* and faid that fuch was his Love, that if he had been poffeffed of 10,000 *l.* he would not leave one Farthing
from

from me. I have been sixteen Years his Widow, and increasing this Fortune by Care and Industry, find upon a true Estimate myself to be worth 2000 *l.* This I communicated to this perfidious Woman, told her, I had concealed my Daughter from the World, as long as Prudence directed me, now I would have her to make an Appearance suitable to her Fortune: I will buy her two Silk Gowns, two full Suits of Silk, and a good Stock of Linen. I can make her a Fortune of 2000 *l.* and she shall appear as such: Then I am sure to surprize the World with a Beauty that they were Strangers to. You are very right, answered this artful Woman, your Daughter's Beauty and Fortune may deserve a Coach, yet you should have a good Room, for you have not one fit to entertain a Gentleman in. That is very true, answered I, but I intend to make that Stone-hall a good Room, I will put two Sash-windows in it, a Deal-floor, and Wainscot it Chair-height. Said she, I can recommend an excellent Workman to you. Do send or write for him, answered I, for I have Deals that have been laid upon Jests in a Hay-loft these two Years to dry, so have I Nails, Wainscot, and such Timber as will be required to lay under the Fir-deals.

She writ, and according to Order two Workmen came, and begun the Work, made the Sashes, and laid the Floor. A Hind's Wife of mine, that lives in a Cottage just at my House, was in Labour, and the poor Man called me up to sit by his Wife, till he rid for the Midwife: I accordingly did, and raised up this Woman and my Maids to go with me to the poor Woman in Labour, that had not one Neighbour within a Mile but me, and the poor Man had two Miles to ride for the Midwife. After she was delivered of a Son, and the Banquet done, the Morning approached, and we returned Home: I thinking to lie down by my Daughter,
but

but no Daughter was there: I shouted out robbed, murdered, and undone, and raised all the House, but none could give an Account of her. The Carpenter came, and said he could not find his Man, though Search was made, but no Man to be found. In this great Hurry came one of my Men, and told me, That the double Horse and Seat was taken out of the Stable. Then, says this wicked Woman, behold, the Fellow must be the Robber that has been guilty of this Stealth: Your Daughter is ungrateful to the best of Mothers, yet she is your own, you have no more, and she knows you will pardon her, as there is no Help for it.

But the Carpenter answering, said, I rather think you the Traitress, that has committed this Robbery: For this is your own Bastard Son, that you bore to a poor Woman's Husband, he served his Apprenticeship to me, is contracted with a young Woman in our Neighbourhood to be married, although it will be a happy Deliverance to her, to get rid of such a Scoundrel: This is a Scene of Vice and Wickedness! I wondered at the Change of his Behaviour, as I never knew him so long in a House, without giving Disturbance, for he is a turbulent wicked Fellow. I am sure, answered she, he is nothing obliged to you for the Character you have given him. It is a just one, said he, so is it as just, that you had your Education at *London*; a grand Man was at the Expence of it, after you bore this Son, and you was his kept Mistress till his Death, although he had a virtuous fine Lady of his own: What you got of him was in Money, which, to my Knowledge your Son has drawn from you, as you were in great Want before you got this Place. I did not know where you were, till I received your Letter, wherein you desired me not to discover him to be your Son to this Family: But as you have betrayed your Mistress of

all

all that she held dear, I cannot connive with the Treachery.

I told the Man how much I should have been obliged to him, if he had given me this Relation in Time; but as he might have no Apprehension of what has happened I excused him, as what he had then related might save me the enquiring any further after my unfortunate Daughter, whose Ingratitude should disinherit her of every Penny belonging to me, and free me of any further Imposition from that vile impudent Adultress, and infamous Wretch. It being just at the Term, I paid her her Wages, all she had to receive was forty Shillings, and turned her out in an Hour's Time. I charged all my Servants to keep it a Secret, for if the Country got the Alarm of my Daughter's Disgrace, I should be teazed with mercenary Lovers, who would pretend to make Amends for my Daughter's Disobedience, although nothing but private Views may be their Errands: And as I never intended to change my State of Life, I would not be importuned upon any Pretence in that Respect. Added I, As I have kept my Daughter so great a Stranger to the World, they will not know nor suspect any Thing about her.

But when I examined myself, and considered what a hoarding and raking I had been making for so many Years past, and all the Wealth that I was entrusted with, what Good had I done with it: I found so little Comfort, that I thought this was a just Judgment sent down upon me, to chastise me for my Ingratitude to that supreme Being, that had enabled me to do Good, which I had carelessly neglected; and my greater Vanity in keeping my Daughter from conversing with honest Mens virtuous Daughters, because I thought them below her, as they were poor; and to have such a vile Adultress to

taint

taint her Morals, by teaching her to defpife me in feven Years Exercife, and with her Arts and Contrivances to betray my Daughter and me. Now, my Dear, I am fo well affured of your Sincerity, that you will give your Opinion honeftly, which of us, Mother or Daughter, is the greateft Faulter?

I anfwered, That her own Reafons were as juft as mine could be, in remarking her Ingratitude to Heaven; and as this Woman had her Daughter fo long under her Care and Inftructions, might eafily work on her tender Mind, and pre-poffefs her with fuch Ideas, and imaginary Notions, as tended only to enfnare and ruin her: But if this Difappointment be only a Call to remind you of what you had forgot, it may prove a Tract to lead you into the right Road to Life-eternal.

So repeating to her the Mifery that I beheld her Daughter in, and likewife her Repentance: All which I have repeated to you before. Adding, that fhe had not difgraced her in being guilty of committing Fornication, nor Adultery; her Crime fhe had fuffered for, and fhe need not fear her committing it again. This was my Errand to you, nor did I divulge it to my Mafter or his Lady. Then fhe got me in her Arms, and embraced me with Tears of Thanks; and faid, Notwithftanding her great Indifcretion, fhe was not willing to look fo mean in their Eyes, as the Knowledge of it might hazard her. I promifed her I would never fpeak of it to my Mafter or Lady. She asked me how fhe muft get her from the Tyrant. I bid her let a Man and a Horfe be ready at Four o'Clock in the Morning, and I would direct them to her, as there was no fear of a Husband being there to interrupt their Defign. So taking my Hand, fhe kiffed it, and faid, Oh! that my Daughter had thy Wifdom. I anfwered, Had fhe been as long under the Directions

rections of my Lady as I had been, she would not have been so easily seduced. That is certain, said she, I have been the real Cause of all her Misery, and will relieve her out of the Hands of that cruel Tyrant.

So she lighted me into the Room, that I was to lie in, and bid me good Night. She rose, and had Tea made against Four o'Clock. When I came down, she asked me how I slept. I told her very well. But, answered she, I have slept none, for thinking of my unfortunate Child. Her ill Fate will be at an End when you receive her again into your Affections, said I. She had got the Men their Breakfasts before I came down. I desired to be excused, it being rather too soon for my Breakfast; but said, If you will give me a little Tea and Sugar, and a thick Slice of that Short-cake, I will breakfast with your Daughter.

She accordingly did, and we set forward on our Journey: After I had taken Leave of her, and got to this Cottage by Seven o'Clock, I desired the Men and Horses to go to an adjacent Farmer's House, to order Corn and Hay. So I went into the sick Woman's House first, found it in decent Order, and the Nurse rocking the Child in the Cradle. I asked how the Mother had rested, and if she had taken any Food. She answered, No, she has drunk a little of the Posset-drink, and thrown it up again. I went to the Bed-side, to see if she was in rest; she lifted up her Hands and Eyes, and made a Motion to pray for me, as far as I could understand by her muttering, that I had released her of the Child: I bid the Woman set on a Pan. She answered, There is a little Tea-kettle, three Cups and Saucers. I bid her cut some Toasts of the Loaf I had brought, and butter them: Which
she

she did, whilst I went to see the Neighbour, who had just arose out of her Bed.

She seeing me, cried, My Dream is out; for I have had the pleasantest Dream of you, and my dear Mother, all this last Night: Now as you are the first I see in the Morning, it boads good Luck to me. Very good Luck, answered I, for I am come to drink Tea with you this Morning; so come into your next Neighbour's, as I see you have no Fire, and we will breakfast together. She did, and I told her what I had done for her: But the Tears of Joy that she in Transports shed, I never will forget. She could not eat one Morsel; so I gave her the Cake that I brought from her Mother, to eat on the Road.

But let me see your Head, said I. I hope you will drink your Tea first, answered she. No, said I; and then taking off the Bandage, I dressed the Wound, and bid her tie on a large Handkerchief, to keep it warm, and to let it be clean washed before they laid the Salve to it. Then I poured out a Dish of Tea, bid her drink it, and eat some Toast. No, answered she, I am so full of Joy, there is no Room for eating; but let me give it to my distressed Sister, for so we often called each other. She went to give her it, but the poor Creature could not raise herself to take the Tea; I put my Hand under her Pillow, and raised her; she drunk up the Tea, but could not eat one Morsel: She looking wishfully on her Neighbour, said, I hear you have got a Release, (and lifting up her Eyes to Heaven) I hope, so will I, in a little Time, be removed out of all my Troubles: (then turning her Eyes to me) Blessed be thou Messenger of Good to her, in restoring her to the Indulgence of a tender Mother; and of Peace to me in my dying Moments.

I

I got the young Creature dreffed, and fhe gave fome of her old Things to the Nurfe, and charged her to take all the Care of her fick Neighbour that was in her Power. I fee her fairly on Horfe-back, and was at Home myfelf at Breakfaft; my Madam was furprized to fee me, asked if the Widow was ill. I anfwered that fhe had been ill, but was much better. I told her of the Diftreffes of the Bricklayer's Wife, and what I had done for her, in the Prefence of the Doctor, that was at Breakfaft; who faid that I gave a very authentick Account of my Patient. No, Doctor, anfwered my Miftrefs, we give our Affiftance to thofe that are not able to get better; but as there feems to be Danger, vifit you this Patient, and do you give me your authentick Opinion of her Cafe. I will, Madam, anfwered the Doctor, if you will order me a Guide to conduct me to the Houfe. My Lady bid me fend the Servant that had rid before me there.

He accordingly did, and brought back the Doctor's Opinion, which was, That fhe would be dead in lefs than twelve Hours. The Nurfe came the next Day, and told me that fhe fent for the Husband, immediately after the Doctor was gone; yet he did not come till this Morning, when his Wife was dead, and laid upon the Bed-ftead, having no Board. The Carpenter coming in, faid, It would be a blith Sight to us both, were mine as fairly dead as thine is. The old Woman anfwered, You have got as fairly quit of her, for fhe is gone. Joy go with her, faid he. So the two Mifcreants gave a great Shout, in the Prefence of feveral of the Neighbours that were there.

One of the Women bid them not fhout, till they got through the Wood. The Carpenter faid, Was not 40 s. and a dead Wife worth 5 l. which
deferved

deferved a Shout. But, faid fhe, where is the 40 s.
He anfwered, There is Furniture worth 5 l. But,
faid fhe, the Wife is to bury, and the Child to
bring up. O Dame, anfwered he, I have as much
Fir-deal as will make her Coffin; I faw her going, for which Reafon my Friend and I had it ready: He will make it for nothing, and we will have
as many of our own Fraternity as will carry her to
the Church-yard; we will fell the Furniture of each
Houfe, and have a merry Caroufe with the Money.
But who muft take Care of the Infant? anfwered
fhe. It will follow the Mother foon; faid he, come,
I will give any one 40 s. that will quit me of it,
and if it die in a Month they will have the Money.
That is as much as to fay kill it when they are
weary of it, faid fhe. If they kill it, they may
hang for it, and if it dies, there is an End of it,
faid he. The old Woman faid, Give me 40 s. and
the Mother's Clothes to make up into Frocks, and
I will take it. It's a Bargain, anfwered the Father,
I know fhe has not many: I took them away by
Littles, juft as I wanted Money; fo take them, and
the Cradle into the Bargain, and there is the Money, which I borrowed to bury the Mother. So
make you the Coffin, put her in, and nail her
down; then we will go for our Brotherhood to lift
her to the Place of Interment; the Child is gone
to Day, we will cant the Goods To-morrow, and
rendezvous the next Day.

This Woman has had this Infant fix Years, as
fond of it as ever Parent was of their own Child;
fhe was foliciting me to get her into my Mafter's
School, a beautiful young Creature, and declares
that the Father never came to fee whether it was
dead or living.——I could innumerate the Hardfhips that I have feen many poor Women labour
under, by the Oppreffion of churlifh Husbands;
yet none were fuch compleat Tyrants as thefe two.

H h   When

When I thought on the general Behaviour of the
vulgar Sort of Men, my Computation was, that
their Want of Understanding deprived them of the
Virtue of mutual Love, as Want of Decency is
Want of Senfe: They marry for mercenary Views,
or for the Conveniency of gratifying their brutal
Appetites; after which their Wives are no more
than their Vaffals, loath them as they do their
Meat, when they can eat no more: Therefore,
Sir, the Danger that attend a married State, was
the Motive which obliged me to be particularly
cautious how I encountered it; for having conceiv-
ed a very mean Opinion of the lower Herd of Mankind, and refolving never to marry for the Sake of
Fortune, fo that all Men were fo indifferent to me;
that all I wifhed or prayed for, was to do my Duty
in the comfortable State of Life I was in: Therefore making this Refolve not to run the Risk of
my future Peace, which a churlifh Husband might
blaft, by involving myfelf in a contentious Life,
that might endanger my future Blifs, was determined never to marry.

yet, when I received the first Letter from this
Youth, and perused it seriously, I thought it could
not be the Language of a savage Breast; nor was
it like the Dictates of a Mechannick, as the Stile
had Dignity in it, which nothing inerior to liberal
Education could support; for in such Places as yours,
we Servants think we have liberal Education at the
Second-hand. This was a Prompter to the lofty
Answer that I returned; which he so far from re-
senting, willingly complied with the seven Years
Injunction, with such Serenity, Wisdom, and Deportment, as justly intitles him to the Prize, that
is not worthy the Pains he has taken for it: But
my Hero down on his Knees, and said, It was an
hundred-fold Reward.

But

But my worthy Master taking him by the Hand, said, Rise, no more Penance, your Worth and Sagacity entitles you to her: Her Virtue, Industry, and Integrity will reward all your Labour of seven Years Suspence. She will leave a Specimen of her Care in my Family; her Mistress has surprized me with the Order and Management, having a robust Constitution, good Morals, and an industrious Disposition. We being ignorant of House-keeping, both very young married, and no Parents to direct us in it; my Wife has told me, that such a Servant was a Blessing to us, whose Industry was an Example to the other Servants. As a Reward for her Diligence, Care, and Integrity, I will lett you that Farm, which my honest old Tenant seems to be removing from in a very little Time, at the same Rent, and on the same Conditions that his Predecessors had it.——— Now, added he, I think it would not be amiss for my Wife and me to withdraw, and leave you to your further Determinations, as this seems to be your first Interview, we will not interrupt them any longer in their private Conversation : My dear Lady taking me by the Hand, she thanked me for the Good I had done the Widow's Daughter, in releasing her from Slavery; and turning to my Lover, said, She will reward all the Pains you have taken for her, and will be a daily Blessing, and they immediately, as the Word was spoke, left the Room.

He fell down on his Knees at my Feet, How unworthy am I of this Blessing! Can all this be true, or is it a Dream? Got hold of my Hand and kiss it. I bid him, on Pain of my Displeasure, rise from his Knees, and consider to whom such Adoration was due. He did, and said, You have the Power to command me to do what you please. Then, said I, let me hear no more of these Encomiums

ums, left I fufpect your Sincerity, for I have refolved not to let my Affection have Rule over my
Reafon; neither have I the Vanity to believe myfelf worthy of that Reward, which both my Mafter and Lady have fo bountifully made mention
of: For what have I done, but difcharged my
Duty in the fame Manner every Servant ought to
do, without any private mercenary Views or Intereft. When I acted three Years in the Capacity of
Cook and Houfe-keeper, my Perquifites fupplied
me with Clothes; then advanced to Houfe-keeper
and Lady's Maid, who gave me more Clothes than
I could wear, befides my other Perquifites, which
were confiderable; for as their generous Souls, when
they vifited their Friends or Neighbours rewarded
the Trouble they gave Servants, fo it was returned
to us, and if I had been thrifty might have faved
Money, befides my Wages. A further Benefit intrufted to me was a great and good Example of
their private Charity, which I daily diftributed,
either to fupport Credit or Hunger; thefe are
Chriftian Benefits, to fhew me the right Road to
Heaven: After all I muft receive a Farm by my
Mafter, which the Tenants that poffeffed it for fo
long a Term of Years, was enabled to live as repu-
tably as any of their neighbouring Freeholders; and
in the Liberality of my Miftrefs's Bounties, which
I am unworthy of, as I cannot expect to make
any Return.

I acknowledge, anfwered he, that great Souls
are unwilling to receive more Favour than they are
able to return: Yet a Misfortune that happened to
a poor *Italian*, which perhaps may enable me to
eafe fome Part of the Hardfhips you are labouring
under. My Father being fent for, to receive a Sum
of Money from a Gentleman of Fortune, who had
employed him in a Building; this Gentleman's Lady called my Father to give his Opinion of a Spinnet,

net, which this *Italian* had made, and bringing it
over to *England*, in order to fell it for a good Sum,
the Ship was drove by Strefs of Weather on Rocks,
and dafhed to Pieces; the Man being prepared for
the Shock, having his Inftrument fecured in a Fir-
deal Cafe, clofe fealed, that the falt Water could
not get Entrance, and well corded; fo fixing another Cord, which he tied round his Waift, fwam
to Shore with this Spinnet, having the Advantage
of the Wind and Tide: So the Lady told him as
he was a Mechanick, that employed fo many Workmen in various Arts of Handicraft, fhe defired his
Opinion of that Spinnet: I have bid 30 *l.* and the
Man will take no lefs than 50 l. for it.

He on Examination found it to be worth a great
deal more Money than the Man had offered it for;
faid, Madam, it is a great Pennyworth at 50 *l.* The
Italian faid that it was great Neceffity obliged him
to offer it for that, as it was worth 80 *l.* but having no Money to fupport him in a ftrange Place,
was the Reafon of his offering it at fo low a Price.
But the Lady fl-ing into a violent Rage againft
my Father, faid that fhe would have got it for the
Money that fhe bid for it, if he had not been; and,
added fhe, will you give 50 *l.* for it? He anfwered
he would. Then, faid fhe, you fhall have it: A
pretty Scoundrel indeed, that can afford a greater
Price than I can. Madam, anfwered he, this is the
moft curious Piece of Workmanfhip my Eyes ever
beheld, fo beautifully embellifhed both within and
without; befides the Skill in fetting the Strings,
that found fo melodioufly as ravifhes the Ear: In
fhort, Madam, I think it fuch a Mafter-piece of
Beauty and Art, that I would be an unjuft Scoundrel, had I not done it the Juftice it well deferves.
She anfwered, that fhe believed and conjectured that
it was a Contrivance between them, to impofe on
her, and faid, as fhe had found out their Knavery,
they

they should not trick her out of her Money. So he said, Madam, as it is the first Time I was ever taken for a Sharper, I will pay for the Trick, and and be the Sufferer myself, not you Madam, and paid the distressed *Italian* 50*l.* and said, I never bought such a Bargain. This enraged her to scurrilous Language, as Rogue, Villain, Pickpocket, Cheat, &c.

The Gentleman came in in the Midst of her Fury, and demanded the Reason: What Violence, added he, have you offered to my Wife, that occasions this Outrage? My Father told him. O Madam, answered he, you want this beautiful Piece of Musick for nothing: I steadfastly believe that these narrow Souls, that would take so much Advantage on a Person in Distress, they would rob him altogether of the whole, if there were not Punishments for such Crimes. I would have given him 10*l.* more for it, if she had behaved like a Gentlewoman; but as she has not, I would burn it in the Fire to Ashes rather than she should have it. So he desired her to withdraw into her Closet, and solicit Pardon for her calumniating Tongue, and I will endeavour to solicit this injured Gentleman, that I dare to say never received such Reproach before. Sir, answered she, I suppose every pitiful Mechannick must be greater in your Esteem than I am. If you behave in this Manner it will be so, Madam, said he. Taking her by the Hand, to lead her out of the Room, she gave my Father such a Buffet with her double Fist, that she burst his Mouth.

The Gentleman more angry, turned her out of the Room, and closed the Door after her, ordered Water to be brought for my Father to wash the Blood off his Face: He gave the *Italian* five Guineas, and begged my Father's Pardon for his Wife's Beha-

Behaviour: My Father begged his, for being the innocent Author of all the Difturbance, and faid, It is only the Lady's Paffion, I hope fhe will harbour a more favourable Opinion of me, after her Paffion is abated. So taking his Leave of the worthy Gentleman, who he faw very much afflicted with the ill Behaviour of his Wife.

The *Italian* hired a Horfe for himfelf, and another Man and Horfe to carry the Spinnet, came Home with my Father, and is with him now, nor does intend to leave him. Now, as I have fome Hope that you will be mine, I hope your Lady will do me the Honour to accept of this Spinnet, for this worthy Father of mine has given it to me. So, anfwered I, you durft not venture this Prefent to my Lady, till you were fecured of me. Yes, faid he, if it was ten Times the Value; but then it would not be from you, before you be mine. Sir, anfwered I, your Wifdom exceeds mine; fo does your Generofity, nor will I refufe you my Hand any longer than Prudence will direct, in departing from this worthy Lady and Mafter. Whofe Goodnefs, he faid, would not keep him much longer in Sufpenfe; and kifs'd my Hand again.

I bid him look what o'Clock it was: Surprized he faid, it was half an Hour paft Eleven, and he thought he had not been half an Hour with me. I faid, your Watch muft be wrong, for my Miftrefs's Bell rings at half an Hour paft Ten. I enquired for the Chamber-maid, and fhe told me that fhe had put her to Bed, and had her Orders to make a Bed for the Gentleman that dined there. I returned, and told him that I was afraid of being difplaced, the Chamber-maid had waited on my Lady. Great Bleffings attend her, anfwered he, for it was parting with my Soul when you went out of the Room. But I told him that we were very

orderly

in sleeping and rising in the Morning. We have no Suppers for Master or Lady, except there be Company, the Servants has cold Meat, Milk, or Beer; if no Strangers, the whole Family is in their Bed by Eleven, and all rises before Six in the Morning. I hope, answered he, you will baulk Sleep one Hour, and oblige me with what is become of the Carpenter's Wife. I said, That I had not delivered my Lady the Commission, her Mother had given me of her Return to her Duty, and likewise the Reformation that the Daughter made of her Mother; for she told me, that as soon as she lighted from her Horse, entered the House, and beheld her Mother, she fainted, and lay within one Minute of an Hour, although all Means seemed to no Effect of bringing her to Life: But the Hind's Wife having two Leaches, let one on each Hand, which after biting, she recovered Life, to the great Joy of her Mother, and all the Family of the Servants.

Her Mother taking her by the Hand, said, "Is this my Daughter who was lost, and is found again; she was dead, and is alive," and has forgot all her Sorrow, as she has received her Child. O my dear Mother, answered she, can you forgive Ingratitude of this Nature, and fainted again; so they laid her into Bed, and as soon as she came out of the second, gave her some Harthorn Drops in Water, and she drinking some of it and got a Sleep: After which she became so much refreshed that she got up, and said, I hope I shall not make another Elopement from my Blessings. Her Mother charged her not to mention what was past, but to think of her future State. O dear and best of Mothers, said she, lay up no more Treasure on Earth, where Moth, Rust, Thieves, &c. break through and steal; but lay Treasure up as our worthy Landlord does in Heaven, where you will not be robbed of it:

What

What Numbers that heavenly Pair relieves is wonderful, the daily Prayers the Poor makes reach Heaven; and although you are not fo able as to do fo much Charity, yet according to your Abilty, no more is required. You need not fear me deceiving you again, for I have got a full Trial of Mankind, and furely the Man will never fee me more, that has ufed me fo cruelly; who, although we were married, he had made fuch Vows to another, as no Marriage could diffolve.

He faid he did not love me, married me for nothing but my Fortune, which his curft Mother perfwaded him to: He curft her to her Face, turned her out of the Cottage, and fhe has not been heard of fince. But, added fhe, I might have been as miferable in another Match, for I think myfelf no longer his Wife, that has made Vows to another.

She bore a Son, which is above five Years old, and the Father never faw him, nor her fince he cut her Head. Her Mother cannot perfwade her to wear a Silk Gown, Lace, Ribbons; yet fays that fhe is more beautiful than ever. She begged of her Mother to get fome Directions from me of Salves and Phyfick, that fhe might do her poor Neighbours good. They fay her Son is the Picture of his Mother.

As I had her Leave, I have told Part of the Story, but thought it too long to conclude; fo if you will go to reft, you may rife in the Morning, and ride with me to vifit the Sick. He faid he was not fleepy, but as it was my Requeft, he obeyed it. The Chamber-maid fhewed him his Bed. I arofe the next Morning at my ufual Hour, but my Lover being up before me, had my Saddle fixed on my little Pad, and his own Horfe being ready, we rode away, all the Servants being entire Strangers to the

I i

Affair

Affair, except the Cook. He gave Charity to every one of my Patients, but did it so secretly that I did not know till the next Day, when they all told me, and prayed for him.

When we got Home, who should salute my Hero, but the Priest, that came to let my Master know that his old Tenant was dead. I went to dress my Mistress, and told them of the Death of the Tenant. Then, said my Mistress, the last honest Man of a worthy Family is gone; and said likewise that she would advise me to marry that ingenious young Man directly, and enter on the Farm: Come I'll plead for the young Man, that you have tortured so long for the Crime of others. I told them, that what they desired in that Respect, I with Pleasure complied to. So my Master went to speak to the Parson, and I told my Mistress the Remainder of the Widow's Story; likewise the little Battle of the Spinnet, which he had reserved to present to her, and the Remark that he made. She said, If I should hasten your Wedding, you will say that I want the Spinnet; for there is nothing that I should covet so much as a Curiosity of that Kind. She went to Breakfast, and my Master told her that they had been perusing his Tenant's Will, who had made him his sole Executor, having no Relation: He said that he would bury him as a Relation, for as he was the Remains of two honest worthy Servants, which are more valuable by much than some Relations; I therefore will shew the Respect due to such in his Interment, for my Mother's Family Vault is in that Church, and he shall be buried in it: All my Tenants shall have Scarves, Hatbands, and Gloves, and likewise all the credible Men in the Neighbourhood.

He gave the Minister Orders for an Account to be taken of every poor Family in the Parish, sent

for

for his Steward to make out a Lift of all his Tenants, with Orners for Silk, Gloves, Hatbands, and Cloaths for the Deceafed's Servants. My Mafter and Lady went into Mourning fix Weeks for him: They diftributed 200 l. amongft the poor Houfholders in the Parifh. The Coffin was ordered to be covered with Black, which my Hero had the Direction of.

After the Minifter and he had got their Inftructions, they immediately fet about getting all Things in Order: The Cook had Orders to prepare a cold Table for the whole Company, we having killed a Beef, fent two large roafting Pieces, the Farmer having left Plenty of Hams, Turkeys, Ducks, Chickens, Butter, Flour, Cheefes, &c. The third Day the Corpfe was to be buried, I went with the the Silk, Gloves, and Hatbands. After all was over, my Mafter ordered the Steward to pay off all the Servants Legacies, and gave me Orders not to leave the Houfe till the Steward came away: Opening the Place where the Money and Securities lay, we found 550 l. 3000 l. on Lands, and 500 l. in Bonds. The Steward fays, There is Corn and Cattle that will raife a fine Sum of Money. He paid the Servants their Wages and Legacies: Is there no mehtion of his wearing Apparel in his Will? faid the Steward; yet you (to the Servants) need not fear getting it, or Part, for I will inform my Mafter of it.

They came and told the Steward one wanted to fpeak to him: When he returned, he faid to me, We are invited to fup with a Relation of mine in this Neighbourhood, who has fent a fingle Horfe Chair for us, I hope you will go with me. With all my Heart, anfwered I, the People are Strangers to me here. So putting on my riding Habit, got into the Chair, and he drove me to the Houfe
which

which I fufpected, although I did not let him
know the leaft Tittle of what happened. My Lover handed me out of the Chair with as noble an
Air and as polite as any Baronet, conducted me into
the Room, and prefented me to his Father, who
faluted me with a modeft Grace, and faid, Thrice
welcome to my Houfe, thou Glory of thy Sex.
What, fays the Steward, has her Fame reached fo
far as here? Ask your Coufin how long it is fince
her Virtues fhined here. Ask me no Queftions in
that Refpect, for there is an Embargo on my Tongue;
therefore excufe me fpeaking on that Subject of
Fame: But (turning to his Father) if you will let
the *Italian* give us a Tune on the Spinnet till Supper be ready; for I believe that this will be the laft
Night you will have it. He anfwered, that it was
his own, he might difpofe of it as he pleafed; and
added, That all Sorrow was departed at the Approach of this worthy Woman, and therefore entertain her as agreeably as you poffibly can: If you
like Mufick, Madam, I will join with you. I
thanked him, and faid, That the Spinnet was all
the Mufick my Lady admired, and that fhe had
taught me to join in Concert, and was Miftrefs of
many Leffons of *Italian* Time, of which I could
do a fmall Matter, although fcarce worth your
hearing.

My Lover had the Man and Spinnet in a Moment in the Room, and as foon as it was uncover-
ed, I was ftruck with Admiration at the Beauty of
it; and faid, This Inftrument pleafes the Eye fo
much, that it cannot offend the Ear. The Artift
made me a Bow, and thanked me for my Approbation on the Mafter-piece of his Art; adding, that
I was the fecond Lady that had feen it in *England*.
I feeing no more Women but the Maid and myfelf;
faid, I hold a Wager that the next Lady that fees
it, will be the beft of the three; as we have feen
it,

it, let us hear it. He begun a Leſſon, and he and me joined the Inſtrument with vocal Muſick, which they all ſaid was well done. Supper being ready, we ſat down, and after Supper the old Gentleman asked if I would chuſe another Tune. But I ſaid, I have been held a little buſy this Day, and beſides you have heard my beſt. Nay, ſaid he, we don't much admire your *Italian*, a good Hornpipe or Volunteer, we could Form a better Judgment on. I anſwered, I might thank my dear Lady for the ſmall Matter that I knew of Muſick. A worthy Teacher, anſwered he, their Tenants live better than ſome Landlords, and this worthy old Neighbour of ours, that is now laid in the Duſt, did more Good out of his Farm, than ſome of our neighbouring Eſquires does out of their great Fortunes. Indeed, anſwered the Steward, I think every Tenant covets to be under him, for there has been 40 about this Farm, that bids me but ask what Rent I would have; but I told them, that I muſt conſult my Maſter firſt.

One wiſer than the Reſt, ſaid he would go to the Fountain-head, and abrudtly asked my Maſter what Rent he would take for the Farm, his Tenant had left. My Maſter told him that it was diſpoſed of: He ſeemed not to be ſatisfied with the Anſwer, and ſaid if he had lett it to the beſt Bidder, he might have got double the Rent. That may be Friend, but will not a Tenant have a better Bargain at the ſame Rent? Certainly, anſwered the other. But if the Farm be diſpoſed of, ſaid the Steward, it is to the Prieſt or your Son; for there has not been a Soul with the Eſquire ſince the old Man died, but theſe two; ſo I am apt to think the one of them will get it.

My Lover and I both bluſhed. What, ſays the Steward, do you both bluſh? You have had a very
expeditious

expeditious Courtſhip, or a very cunning one; for I heard my Maſter bid the Prieſt come to his Houſe, and bring a Licenſe to marry a Couple. You are jeſting, ſaid I. I am not upon my Word, anſwered he. The old Gentleman ſaid to the Steward, You call this a ſudden Wedding, but my Son will not call it ſuch: This fair one put ſeven Years Trial of his Skill to gain her, which ſet forth his Wiſdom; as for Cunning he is above it. The News, anſwered the Steward, is as welcome to me as you: I am proud of the Thoughts of this unkind wiſhed for Relation, that has kept me a Stranger to what would have given me and mine much Pleaſure to have known, for it was my Opinion ſhe would not marry any Man: I thought ſhe had been a Man-hater, for ſhe was ſo often complaining of bad Huſbands; yet it ſeems you have found out the Way to her Heart.

I begged his Silence: I have done, anſwered he, my Couſin and me will be Bed-fellows to Night, perhaps he may have a ſtrange one To-morrow Night, but I will name no one. Nay, ſaid I, Stewards may ſay what they pleaſe to Tenants, leſt if the Rent be not ready they drive their Cattle. But (turning to the old Gentleman) Sir, I am very ſure it is paſt your Time for Reſt, the Clock has ſtruck Ten. He anſwered, that Eight was his Time ſince his Indiſpoſition: So ſaluting me, bid me Goodnight. His Son handed him to his Room, who preſently came back. The Steward ſaid, Come let us be no longer upon the Banter, keep me no longer in the Miſt, but be frank, as it will not be in your Power to keep it much longer.

He ſaid, Get Leave of my Darling. I anſwered, You have my Leave to inform your Couſin of what he ſeems deſirous to know. So beginning with the Courtſhip, concluded with my Maſter's offering
him

him the Farm. In Troth, faid the Steward, Coufin, if you have had a hard Courtſhip, you feem to make a very happy Conclufion in the Profpect of a good Wife and a good Farm. He told him, that he intended to make a Prefent of the Spinnet to my Miftrefs. So you may, anfwered he, if it was worth 100 *l.* yet, in my Opinion, nothing under the Sun would fit her Tafte more: Therefore let it be packed up in the Morning, fend this *Italian* to my Houfe with it, and after the Grace is faid, prefent my Lady with it. Well, anfwered I, now you feem to have tranfacted what is to be done, I therefore will be obliged to the Maid if ſhe will ſhew me where I am to fleep, which ſhe did.

I rofe the next Morning at my ufual Hour, and after I was dreffed, went into the Parlour, where was the Steward and his Coufin: The Steward faid, This Man is as much afraid of approaching you as if you were a Dutchefs; he ftands in greater Awe than ever a Lover did on the Wedding-day. As he is fo very humble a Servant, anfwered I, it is to be hoped he will not be a proud Mafter. No, anfwered he, I rather chufe to be all Obedience, Love, and Duty, telling me, that he had fent the Spinnet and the Artift with it, and that the Prieft were to breakfaft with us at the Farmer's Houfe. Leaving my Compliments to the old Gentleman, the Chair being ready, the Steward drove me to the Farm-houfe, where the Prieft was waiting, who handed me out, and welcomed me Home again. Sir, I thank you, anfwered I, but muft foon quit this Home, and return. Now, fays the Steward, was not I right. Come, no more Banters before Breakfaft, faid I. Seeing the Houfe in very good Order, I faid to the Maid, Wilt thou like being a Servant to my Lady? Very well, anfwered ſhe. So I hired her to ferve the Cook.

As soon as Breakfast was done, we set forward on our Journey; my Lover came up to us in a new Suit. Said the Priest to the Steward, in such a Whisper that I heard, Is this the Bridegroom? It is very likely, said the other. Then, said the Priest, I am sure of getting as good a Neighbour as I have lost. So the merry Priest was all Mirth, which made the Journey seem shorter. As the Clock struck Eleven, we arrived; my Lady came to me, welcomed me, and bid me come up Stairs, for she had something of Importance to say to me. When I came into the Dressing-room, there was a new Silk Gown, a Pair of her Stays, Shoes, Stockings, and every Particular. Now, said she, I will send the Chamber-maid to help you to dress, and pray be expeditious, for you must not exceed the canonical Hour.

She went down into the Room to my Master, the Priest, and my Lover, and said to him, Young Man, you are going to receive the Hand of this Woman, whose Price far exceeds Rubies, and as you have been a dutiful Servant to your adopted Father, I hope you will be an affectionate Husband to her: It is not the Interest of any Family to part with such a faithful Servant; yet they must be mercenary that would desire to deprive the World of such a Pattern, as I am well assured she will be. He paid her Reverence, and said, he was unworthy of so fine a Woman; but what he fell short of her Merit, hoped to make up with Diligence and Affection. She answered, that she verily believed it.

The Priest added, that no young Man had so general a good Character in his Parish. And, says my Master, I think him a worthy Fellow, and you will find her as good a Neighbour, and as con-
stant

ftant a Communicant as any in your Flock: But, Sir, in examining the Will of the Deceafed, I find he hath left you a Legacy of 100 *l.* and mentions, that as your Salary was flender, it was in my Power to advance that Sum, which to me feemed as if he repented he had not bequeathed you more. Pray, Sir, inform me what Salary does the Rector give you? Forty Pounds a Year, anfwered the Prieft. And no Church Fees? faid my Mafter. None at all, Sir, anfwered the Prieft; all the Fees goes into the Rector's Pocket. How can you, Sir, maintain your large Family, a Wife, five Daughters, and a Servant out of that? I keep no Servant, anfwered he; my Wife obliges her Daughters to Induftry by her Example, otherwife it would not do. Indeed when our Children were young, my Wife could not do without a Servant; but no fooner could the eldeft keep the youngeft, but fhe difmiffed her Servant, and performed the Office of a Servant-maid herfelf, finding my Circumftances obliged her thereto, or otherwife run behind-hand in the World. I think, anfwered my Mafter, that I have heard that the Rector did no Duty, except one Sermon a Year: Is it true? Very true, Sir, anfwered he. Then, faid my Mafter, as you have the full Charge of the Flock, the Sick to vifit, the Dead to bury, and the Living to admonifh, your Rector ought to give you better Share of the Revenue: For better is he that is fcorned, and has a Servant, than he that is honoured, and has none: Is not the Labourer worthy of his Hire? You are obliged to keep a Horfe out of this fmall Salary, and when you are called out of your Bed to baptize a weak Child, or adminifter the Sacrament, pray, Sir, who gets you your Horfe ready? Sir, faid he, I having often Midnight Duty to do, and the Parifh being large, whenever I am called upon that Duty, fo good a Wife have I, that fhe has my Horfe ready faddled for me, whilft I am dreffing my-

felf

felf. My Mafter faid, I think it fo great a Hardfhip that a Minifter of the Gofpel fhould be fo ftraightened in his Circumftances, as not to be enabled to keep a Servant, that I think myfelf bound in Duty to fupport that Want, by paying you the Legacy, and adding 50 *l.* to each of your Daughters and Wife, which will amount to 300 *l.* more: The Intereft of which Money will enable you to keep a Servant, and make a fmall Provifion for your five Daughters.

The Prieft amazed at the Bounty of his great Benefactor, made a reverend Bow, and begun a Speech of Thankfulnefs and Gratitude; but was forbid to proceed, by that worthy Gentleman, who told him, he knew he was going to pay him more Homage than he wanted to receive; and you will oblige me more if you will give this young Man a matrimonial Lecture, that is going to enter into a conjugal State.

In the Interim my Lady came up, and told me what had paffed; adding, how much fhe was grieved to hear a Minifter of God affert, that he had no more to maintain his Family but 40 *l.* a Year, which was not fufficient for Food, exclufive of Raiment; but your worthy Mafter will eafe that Yoke. Pray let me examine your Drefs:—Indeed, Mrs. Bride, I think you have compleated the Quaker. Don't you think it grand for a Carpenter's Bride, anfwered I, Madam? Although a Mechanick, fays fhe, he has the Accomplifhments of a Gentleman; but here he comes with your Mafter, and the Prieft, who faid, The Time is run out to the laft Quarter of an Hour. Well, anfwered my Mafter, the Bride, and her Maid (pointing to my Miftrefs) are ready, and the Chapel-door is open, fo let us enter. He took me by the Hand, led me into the Chapel, attended by my Miftrefs, Prieft,

and

and Bridegroom, and the Grace was quickly dif-
patched.

When we entered the Dining-room, the *Italian*
and the Spinnet was there, which my dear Lady
obferving, faid, Here is a moft beautiful Inftrument.
Indeed fo it is, anfwered my Mafter. Says the Prieft,
I never beheld fo great a Curiofity. Who is the
Owner of this Matter-piece of Art? faid my Miftrefs. I, Madam, anfwered the Bridegroom, and
hopes that your Goodnefs will accept of this fmall
Mite in Token and Acknowledgment of ten-fold
Value received. If it founds as well as it looks, I
will thankfully accept it. The Artift gave an *Italian*
Leffon, that my Lady faid was as great a Ravifher
of her Ear as it was to her Eye: Said, It was a Prefent too great to accept. But I told her, that there
was a Reward already received.

After Dinner, my Lady had provided Gloves for
all my Fellow-fervants, who were furprized, never
hearing of, nor fufpecting a Lover.——Then my
Lady bid the new Houfe-keeper come in, who was
weeping, and faid, What Happinefs fuch a Prefident gave the Family. She deferves every Thing
that thou haft faid, anfwered my Lady; fo does thy
grateful Acknowledgments deferve every Thing that
fhe has done in improving thy Knowledge. She
therefore delivers up all her Truft to thee, in whom
I place the fame Confidence I did in her: Therefore, as fhe has done by you, do you by others; fo
dry up all your Tears, for I rejoice that fhe will
make a good Wife to a worthy Man that was dying for her, I hope fhe will produce fome Copies
of herfelf, and that it advances you to her Station,
your Sifter to yours, and as fhe has hired one in
your Sifter's Place, I hope you will take the fame
Pains to inftruct her, as has been taken with you,
by which Means her Order will be continued in my
Houfe.

Houfe. I would be very unhappy to fee fuch Confufion, and have the fame Reafon of Complaints of
bad Servants that others have, neither have I a Conftitution to buftle and braul with fuch: So as I
gave her, I give you a Guinea, her Wages and Perquifites you may likewife expect, the Indulgence
fhe had, if you deferve it, as I hope you will.

Then I delivered to her the feparate Notes of all
my Charge of Sets of Table and Tea China, of all
Glaffes, Salvers, and every feparate Item belonging
to Deferts; of all the Stock of Sweet-meats wet
and dry, Pickles, Hams, Tongues, and Bacon-flitches;
of the Bed and Table Linen. There is my Book of
daily Provifion, containing Ducks, Geefe, Turkeys,
Chickens, Pullets, Capons, Beef, Mutton, Lamb,
and Veal: So is there the Book of Confumption,
which gives an Account of every individual Fowl
that was bought, and when it was dreffed for the
Family Ufe; as well as every feparate boiling, roafting, ftewing, or baking Piece of Beef, likewife e-
very Joint of Mutton, Lamb, or Veal, for thefe
nine Years paft, which the Notes the Steward has
filed in his Office confirm the Truth of.

So can I juftify the Juftice of this Servant, (meaning the new Houfe-keeper) that has not impaired
you of one fingle Fowl or Chicken by Neglect or
Injuftice thefe feven Years, which is more than I
can fay for myfelf; for befides the Lofs of fo much
Poultry fed into Difeafes by my Ignorance, the impairing of your Health was a far greater Crime, as
you had fuch fent to your Table, which I am very
well affured deftroyed your Health: But as foon as
I was directed the right Way, I never left it, nor
has fhe ever had a fick or diftempered Fowl fince
that Time. I feeing her Care, Induftry, and Capacity, defired the School-mafter to teach her Writing
and Book-keeping, which fhe readily obtained, and
has

has for thefe two Years paft been as bufy in acting
the Houfe-keeper as the Cook. Although fhe did
not believe me, never feeing a Man in my Company,
I told her that fhe one Day was to rife a Step high-
er. I let her into my Method, by which fhe can
act in the Manner I have before related. Having
nothing more but the moft material Part, *viz.* all
your wearing Apparel, Linen, and Jewels'; fo giving
her the Lift of them, my Lady defired to fee it, and
after fhe had looked it over, would return it her a-
gain.

My Miftrefs bid me go with her into her Room,
where fhe opened her Efcrutore, and taking out the
Note of her wearing Apparel, faid, Behold the
Marks there made at the feparate Articles, which I
have put into a Box, which is nailed, and clofe
corded down, left you fhould make a Diftribution
before you leave the Houfe: Therefore make another
Lift, and leave out all that you fee the Mark fet on,
and in the mean Time I will go and get another
Leffon on the Spinnet, which charms me very much.
She accordingly did, and juft as I had finifhed the
Copy, fhe came into the Room, and faid, You
have finifhed it. Yes, Madam, faid I, and wonders
what I muft do with fuch Stocks of Apparel as
you have packed up for me, as I intend to wear
very little but Home-fpun Gowns in the Country.
If you won't wear them, keep them for your Daughters, tell them they were the Reward of virtuous
Induftry, and the beft deferving fhall have moft of
them: This will fpur up your Daughters Induftry,
for fine Clothes are a great Temptation to young
Creatures. You fmile at me, added fhe, but I have
made your Mafter, Prieft, Bridegroom, and *Italian*,
laugh at your Books of Provifion and Confumption,
and your Mafter declares he will have all your nine
Years Notes compared with the Provifion Book,
to fee how they agree the one with the other.

The

The Steward was ordered to pay the Bridegroom 100 *l.* for his Bride's ten Years Service, and 21 *l.* for the Interest. The Bridegroom said, that he would receive none of it, as he was indebted double the Sum. My Master said, You shall have it seven Years without Interest, in which Time I don't at all dispute but by your own Industry, and the Assistance of a good Help-mate, will enable you to pay it with Ease and Pleasure at the Expiration of that Time; as you had no Hopes ten Days since of this Marriage, I conjecture that you have not given proper Notice to those who have your Money upon Interest to pay it in. He answered, Having no need of it, did not call it out of the Hands it was in; yet I think six Months Notice is what is common in such Cases, and it being near *Martinmas,* I intend giving Warning to pay it against *May.* But that will not answer your present Demand, said my Master, for your Father designs to put you in Possession of his Trade and Business, to give up House, and board himself and his three Sons with you, he finding himself unable to undergo his former Fatigue, resolves to pass the Remainder of his Days in Peace: Then will you have his Stock of Timber, that he employed his neigbouring Journeymen to work in the Winter Quarter; when he could not build, he kept them employed in making Houshold Furniture. This was an Act of Humanity to those poor Men, that have Families, which I hope will give you the same Pleasure it has done your honest Predecessor: Besides as you have so great an Artist as this Gentleman, (pointing to the *Italian*) that is so well pleased with your Family, he, no doubt, will instruct you in his Curiosity, which may be of Advantage to you; so that if you want 2 or 300 *l.* more, you may have it.

My

My deceafed Tenant left me this Money in Truft, which Truft I intend to difcharge in Honour of his Memory. It is my firm Belief he intended this Fortune for a facred Ufe, by the Hint he gave me on your Legacy, Sir, (directing himfelf to the Prieft) which he repenting was fo fmall; told me that I had it in my Power to add to it, which, in Effect, was to fay, If I have not left this Fortune to the righteous Heirs, I will chufe one in whom I can confide in doing Juftice. I intend to apply it in the following Manner, 1000 *l.* of this Money fhall be a Bank Stock, for any Farmer in that Parifh, that appears to want 50 *l.* and ask it as a Charity, to help him to a Stock, or otherwife by Cultivation to improve his Farm; the above Sum paying no Intereft for feven Years, fuch Farmer finding Security to pay it at the Expiration of that Time.

The Remainder of my Tenant's Money, I intend to apply in building a Free-fchool on a Piece of Ground I have very near the Church, and fix two Mafters, the head one to have 40 *l. per Ann.* and the Ufher 10 *l.* who fhall teach all the Children of the Parifh, whofe Parents or Friends apply for this Benefit as a Charity; and as foon as the Weather becomes feafonable for building, a Plan fhall be drawn for a School and Dwelling-houfe for two Mafters, the head Mafter to have eight Rooms, and the Ufher four.

The Prieft anfwered, If the Mafters are elected, I will ftand Candidate. My Mafter faid, That the inftructing of Youth, was, in his Opinion, full as facred as the Pulpit; yet, added he, I don't think there is one Prieft in 100, that can fubject himfelf to confult the Tempers and Capacities of Children. I am that one, anfwered the Prieft, who have a

Specimen

Specimen to indicate, that I have confulted the
different Capacities of Boys and Girls, who differ
as much in Minds as Faces: I have taught my five
Daughters to read, and four of them to write; two
Sons of my Clerks I have inftruƈted to read, write,
and underſtand Accompts, vulgar and decimal, and
one I have taught both the Latin and Greek Authors, and ſomething of the *Hebrew* Language: I
was obliged to have Recourſe to different Methods
with every one of them, in communicating the
Authors and my Thoughts to them; but the eldeſt
delights me in his quick Progreſs, for he takes in
Learning as faſt as I can give it him. How old is
the Youth? ſaid my Maſter. Sixteen, Sir, anſwered
the Prieſt.

My Maſter ſaid, You ſhall be head, and if you
judge the Youth qualified for your Uſher, you
ſhall have it in your Power to put him into that
Poſt, as it will be a Year before the Building is
finiſhed, and fit for a Family to dwell in; during
which Time I recommend to you all poſſible Diligence, in compleating the Boy for his Undertaking.

This worthy Gentleman performed all theſe Cha-
rities: My Husband's Diligence and Pains was ſuch
as enabled him to ſupport his Family with every
Neceſſary of Life, to make all about him happy.
Nay, were the Night a Month long, I could entertain you with this worthy Man's Humanity and
Charity, who built a little Houſe, with four Beds
in it, for any of the Poor, that were afflicted with
Wounds, or Sickneſs; which he ſaid his Wife
would cure, for he was ſure that a Bleſſing attended all her Endeavours. He ſent Home a Hogſhead
of *Jamaica* Sugar, I wondered at ſo large a Quantity of brown Sugar, and asked him what I muſt
do with it. He anſwered, Make Wine of it. I
anſwered,

anfwered, That I never made Wine of coarfe Sugar, but will try if this will anfwer the fame End. He faid, that his Reafon told him that it would; for, added he, all the double-refined Sugars is made from this Drofs, and the Juice of your Fruit will refine it, as well as the Sugar-boilers will do it with the Combuftables. I anfwered, My Dear, you muft be right; and, pray, tell me what is the Expence of this Quantity. He anfwered, that there was a Ton Weight of it, which he got for 18 *l.* Well, anfwered I, then if that be the Cafe, it will not be Two-pence a Pound, which will make a very great Difference from Ten-pence; for I never made any Wines of Sugar under that Price, and as we have a very great Quantity of Fruit this Seafon, the deceafed Batchelor took great Delight in planting all Manner of Fruit Trees.

The Cherries being all full ripe, I fet to work, and got them pulled; after all the Stalks were taken from them, I had 25 Gallons of bruifed Fruit to a Pulp, unto which I put the fame Quantity of Water, and let it ftand 24 Hours, ftirring it well every four Hours: Then I made three Strainers of coarfe thin Linen Cloth, and ftrained all the Liquor through thefe Cloths; after I had fqueezed the Juice out, I put the fqueezed Fruit into the Cloths we put the Cheefes in to prefs, wafhed the Cheefe-prefs clean, I put in the fqueezed Cherries, to prefs all the Juice and Pulp clean out of them, fetting a Tub to receive what drained from it. I then put all the Juice together, and meafured it, of which there was 42 Gallons, to which I put 16 Stone of this Sugar, and ftirring it well, let it ftand 24 Hours, ftirring it well every three Hours. I having a Wine Hogfhead ready, in which there had been *Florence* Wine, I tunned it into it, and had ten Gallons more than it held: I let it have Room to foment out at a Spile-hole, and as foon as it was

done

done working clofed it up. I then fummoned up all my Reafon of Wine-making, in order to make as much Wine of my Fruit as poffible, as I had fuch a large Quantity of Sugar, which I determined to make the greateft Advantage of, as it was the Will and Pleafure of my worthy Husband, which Duty and Love obliged me to obey.

I got my white Currants pulled, bruifed, and ordered in the fame Manner I did my Cherries, and having 12 Gallons of bruifed Berries, I added 12 Gallons of Water; which after ftraining and pref- fing had 22 Gallons of Liquor, to which I put eight Stone of Sugar, and two Pounds of dried Elder Flowers; after it had wrought 24 Hours in this Liquor, ftirring it well every three Hours, I ftrained it through a Hair-fieve, fqueezing out all the Flowers, and tunned it into a Wine Half-hogf- head, and had as much over as filled an eight Gal- lon Cask, all which I let foment as above, and then clofed them up.

The red and black Currants, when gathered and bruifed, had the fame Quantity of Juice, to which I put the fame Quantity of Sugar, and had the like Quantity of Wine.——Of yellow and chriftal Goofeberries mix'd I had 35 Gallons of bruifed Fruit, adding the fame Quantity of Water, and preffed out the Juice, to which I put 24 Stone of Sugar; I let it ftand as before mentioned, and then tunned up a Hogfhead: I had 30 Gallons more, to which I added 30 Pounds of Sugar, and let it ftand 24 Hours, and tunned up a Half-hogfhead of this, and had other four Gallons of it left.

My red Goofeberries when bruifed were 12 Gal- lons, to which I added the fame of Water; after ftraining and preffing them I had 21 Gallons of Li- quor, to which I added eight Stone of Sugar; I
tunned

tunned up a Half-hogfhead, and had eight Gallons more, which I casked up.———I had the fame Quantity of green Goofeberries, of which I made the like of Wine, in the above Manner. When I fummoned up my Stock of Wine, I had two full Hogfheads, five Half-hogfheads, and 46 Gallons in fmall Casks; which had confumed one Half and 30 Pounds of my Ton of Sugar. The Quantity of Sugar that remained I grudged to keep by me, as I thought it would do more Service in the Wine Order: So that as foon as the Brambles were full ripe, I fet as many poor Children to gather, as filled me an open headed Hogfhead full, which when bruifed and divided into two Casks, I added the fame Quantity of Water that I had of bruifed Fruit.

Our Garden being hedged round with large Quicks, which bore Sloes, near the Size of Damfins, which being ripe, we gathered a Bufhel of them, and bruifed them; I added Sugar as Reafon told me that it would give a rough Tafte to the Wine; after it had ftood the above Time, I ftrained and preffed the Fruit, and meafuring my Liquor had 84 Gallons, to which I put 32 Stone of Sugar; which I let ftand the ufual Time, and then tunned it into a Wine Butt, and had 10 Gallons more. After all my Wines were done fomenting, I fecured all their Spile-holes, and clofed them all; as foon as Winter approached I clofed up all the Cellar Windows, and put a great Quantity of Horfe Dung before them, fo that my Wine Celler, in the Middle of Winter, was warmer than any Room in the Houfe.

At *Chriftmas* I faid to my Hufband, My Dear, you never enquire of me how my Wines prove, nor what Quantity I have made. He anfwered, My Life, the Reafon of that is, becaufe you need not a-
ny

ny Supervifor. But you, anfwered I : Therefore go with me into the Cellar, and let us try thefe Wines. I took feven clean Wine Glaffes. He faid, What have you fo many Sorts of Wine? You will fee I have, anfwered I. But when he entered the Cellar he was ftruck with Wonder at the Number of Casks, which were one Pipe, two Hogfheads, five Half-hogfheads, and feven fmall Caks; every Cask having the Name of the Wine, and the Day of the Month when it was tunned writ upon Paper, and pafted upon each End of them: He fpiled all the fmall Casks which were tranfparently fine, fo he took the feven Glaffes full of Wine, and fhewed to the *Italian*, who faid, That after that Wine got Age, it would not be inferior to foreign Wines; for this Wine made of green Goofeberries is tinctured with *Champaigne*, and if it had three Years of Age, it would be more near the Rellifh. That of the Brambles will be very near red *Port*, it has the Colour and rough Tafte, and it will be a very ftrong Wine; for it has a Body that will keep 20 Years. Your white Currant Wine has the Flavour of *Frantoniack*. The Cherry Wine feems to tafte of *French* Wine. Your Goofeberry Wine fweet *Mountain*. The red Goofeberry Wine is flavoured like *Burgundy*. Your red Currant Wine is a very pretty tafted one, give it Age, and you will have great Credit by it.

My Husband faid to him, Sir, go with me into the Wine Cellar, and fee the Quantity of Wine fhe has made; likewife the Care taken to keep it warm. Which they both gave fuch Praife to, as foothed my Vanity. My Husband faid, that he could, by the Virtue of a good Wife, drink Wine cheaper than his Neighbours could Small-beer. But, faid I, pray, Sir, what Neighbour have you, that would give his Wife a Ton of Sugar to make Wine of? It is your great Care and Induftry, that enables

your

your Wife to furnifh your Cellar with Wine, as well as your Table with Meat.——— In fhort, his great Wifdom, Generofity, and Example, juftly entitled him to the Efteem of all that knows him: As I have the Pleafure to be alone with you, tell me as frankly of your matrimonial State, as I have of mine.

I anfwered, that if I had laid up as much Treafure in Heaven as fhe, before I entered into that State, I, no doubt, might have received the Reward that fhe had done; and as I thought myfelf remifs in my Duty, perhaps I got as good a Husband as I deferved: You know I told you before there is many better, many worfe; your Story has ravifhed my Ears, but as there is not the fame Harmony in mine, you fhall not have the Pain of hearing that Part of my indulgent Husband, whofe Affection, Induftry, and Care, may appear if I write out my Hiftory, which may have as many Points of Admiration, in the Recital of my 24 Years hard travelling in one County. Wherein divers Cruelties were committed, by the Power of fome Juftices, whofe Fortunes entitles them to get a Commiffion of the Peace; for there is no Enquiry after Morals, Integrity, or Wifdom.

I fuffered a ten Years Perfecution by the Tyranny of one of thofe mifcreant Heroes, that laboured very hard to rob me of the Profit of my lawful Endeavours; three Years he laboured againft my Character without Succefs: I petitioned Heaven to witnefs my Innocence, and he that does turn the Hearts of Men as feems beft with his infinite Goodnefs and Wifdom, feemed to interfere in my Caufe, which was as follow. This Tyrant by the Suggeftion of a cunning Aunt, laid a Snare for my Character, and when a very proper Opportunity offered, having an Affize Trial, called my Husband to

him

him, and faid, The Judge bid me tell you to pro-
vide for him and the Family, for he will be at your
Houfe; befides the Chancellor, and many of the
Council: And, with all feeming Refpect, bid him
make free of his Cellars, for *French* Wine, or any
Thing in his Houfe to do him Service.

My Husband, with all the Refpect due to fo
much Humility and good Neighbourhood, thanked
his Worfhip, and came Home, and told me. I anfwered, that I hoped he would be a better Neighbour than his Aunt, that lived next Door to me
nine Years, and was very often a Borrower, but
had very little to lend; I have fupplied her with fat
Ducks, Chickens, Bacon, Butter, Bread: If I got
lean Fowls for my fat, I was well off; Bread, Butter, or Bacon, they were above taking Notice to
pay, it was the Servants that borrowed in the Miftrefs's Name, and I am apt to think for her Ufe,
as I had Part of her Entertainments to fupply when
fhe had Company. She having a great Pleafure in
entertaining thofe above her Rank and Circumftances after fhe got Riches, but hated the Sight of
all thofe that were her greateft Benefactors in the
Time of her Diftrefs; and if this be real Kindnefs
offered to you from her Nephew, it is a Gratifica-
tion to me for a Service I did him, before he was
Mafter of this great Fortune.

When he was a Scholar about 18 Years of Age,
he came from the Univerfity to pay a Vifit to his
Friends; his Aunt's Houfe was his Home, I being
her next Door Neighbour, having a well accuftomed Inn, a Servant told me that one wanted me in
the Entry, and when I came there, who was it but
this young Youth, who very complaifantly enquired
after my Health. I thanked him, and welcomed
him into the Country. He faid, I have a Horfe
to fell you. I anfwered, I have no Manner of Skill
in

in buying Horfes, my Husband makes thefe Bargains. But this is a wooden Horfe for drying Linen on, faid he. I anfwered, Sir, my Husband fupplies me in thofe Articles. But, faid he, this Horfe is mine, and I want to fell it. I at that Inftant beheld a Blufh, and obferved a Cloud in his Brow, frankly faid, Pray, Sir, tell me the Price of this Horfe? He anfwered, A Crown. So I gave it him, but at the fame Time faid, I had not the leaft Occafion for it, but to oblige him. He returned me Thanks, and affured me that it was a very good Horfe, and would fend it up by one of his Aunt's Servants.

He fent it me, and to my Surprize this Horfe had fcarce a Leg to ftand upon; my Husband in great Fury asked me what I had bought that rotten Stick for. I anfwered, Only for Billet Wood, and to oblige a Youth that muft be pinched for Pocket Money: As his Aunt hath long Fetches, this feems to me to be one of them, for I never fpoke to the young Man, nor had the leaft Acquaintance of him; yet I faw in his Countenance that if I expected his future Notice, I muft buy the Horfe, as he was defigned by his Aunt for this great Fortune, which you fee he hath accomplifhed, and if there be the leaft Gratitude in him he will not forget that Crown for this rotten Stick, which was not worth Twopence.

However the Chancellor coming to our Houfe, called for fome *French* Wine, and faid, it was not good: My Husband fent to borrow fix Bottles of this great Man's Wine, telling the Chancellor whofe Wine he had borrowed for him. But one of the Council lodged at this great Man's Houfe, who had bid the Lawyer make Enquiry of his Brethren after fix Bottles of Wine, which he made a Prefent of to the Council: This Agent in the Prefence of the

Judges

Judges and Council, which dined all together at *Carliſle*, enquired of the Chancellor how he liked the Wine that was ſent him to the Inn from Eſquire *Flaſh*. He ſaid, I had no Wine but what I paid the Landlord for, who told me he borrowed it of him. At which a Rumour of Infamy was raiſed by the Judges and Lawyers, who determined never to come to this Inn again.

This Lawyer writing a Letter full of Invectives to this Antagoniſt, who took the Opportunity at a Banquet, after the Lady's Recovery of a Child-bearing, when he had a full Drawing-room; amongſt whom was a worthy Gentleman and a great Benefactor to this Inn of ours, in whoſe Name he ſent a Servant, deſiring my Husband to come and ſpeak with them, who had ſomething of Conſequence to communicate to him. My Husband full of Joy told me the Meſſage that he had received, which he verily believed was that theſe Gentlemen were about ſetting forward Horſe Races; which, added he, will give ſome Relief to the great Loſs that we have lately received.

So full of Expectation went to the Houſe of this great Man, who, as ſoon as he had entered his Drawing-room, roſe up, and having the Lawyer's Letter in his Hand, ſaid, Here, Villain, is thy Character in black Lines; ſure no Gentleman of Credit will ever frequent the Houſe of a common Robber: Villain! I will bring thou to a dry Morſel, for robbing me of my Wine, for which I ſhall bring thy Houſe unto Deſolation.———Nor did you ever ſee a Man in ſuch Diſtraction as my Husband came Home to me in, ſaid, That if he had robbed this Hero of 1000*l.* on the Highway, he could not have called him more Rogues, or Villains: Yet, added he, I can call my ſacred Judge to witneſs, that I never wronged the World of Six-pence, to
my

my Knowledge. For what did he call you such Names? said I. For his six Bottles of Wine, said he, which he denieth that he lent me; he has got a Letter from some of the Counsellors, which he threateneth Destruction to my House with, for he swears to shew it to every one of my Guests, until I be brought to Beggary. But did you receive all this Calumny with Silence? Had you not Courage to justify your Innocence? He said, That the Surprize and Disappointment struck me into such a Heat, that I remained dumb for some Minutes, my Tongue stuck fast to the Roof of my Mouth, until I heard the Voice of my worthy Benefactor, who said, Hast thou nothing to speak in thy own Justification? If thou art innocent speak for thyself; but if thou art guilty I am sorry for thou; and am afraid that thou wilt be ruined. I begun to tell the whole Story to this Gentleman, but was interrupted by the Aunt and Lady with Rogue! and Villain! for daring to justify myself in their Presence, who thought proper to condemn me. But, said I, take a Witness with you to the Steward, who you told me was with his Master that very Day the Judges left thy House, when you offered him Pay for this Wine, in the Presence of this Steward, who, I hope is more worthy than his Master, but if I should be deceived, and he deny your offering to pay him on that Day, it will be a very hard Task for you to clear your Innocence of this Aspersion, which that Slanderer is so eager in smiting your Character with.

He took an honest Man with him to the Steward's: But what an Extacy of Joy did I receive, when they told me how far the Steward exceeded his Master in Humanity and Justice; for when my Husband told him the Treatment that he had received, he was very sorry, but said, it was lucky that he was present when he came to pay for the Wine, that Day the Judges went from his House; adding,

that

that such was his Opinion of his Honesty, if he had not come on that Day, he should have thought him as clear in Fact: But, added he, how my Master could use an honest Man in that Manner, surprizes me.

All this was not sufficient to give my Husband Peace of Mind; he could not sleep, nor would let me sleep, still ruminating on his House being brough to Ruin, by the Malice and Power of his unjust Adversary. I bid my Husband fear that great Being, that sets out a Tyrant's Limitation, and disables him from exceeding his Boundary: The Infamy was hard to bear, but would not the Guilt have been much harder; therefore give God the Praise of an honest Heart, which your Antagonist wants: Although you have your Foibles, you might be more diligent, careful, and affectionate in your Family; but that is to me, not to the World, which, I dare say, you never did Wrong to. As to this great Man I will write him a Letter in the Morning, and shew how much I love or fear him; nor will I tamely let him rob me of my Character, nor will be willing to let my Children be branded with their Father's stealing this Tyrant's Wine.

By Three in the Morning I arose, and writ him a Letter, the Contents of it were, How much the warm Reception had terrified my Husband, but how little it had frightened me, who gave him the Consolation of his Worship's committing the same Mistake on a far greater Man, whose Light so shines that Thousands seeth his good Works and praises them; whose Lady never joined in Concert against a Person in Distress: Adding, that if this alworthy Man met with the same Fate from his Worship, what Reason my Husband had to be content with his, and if he sollicits his Judge, he will relieve

his

his Wrongs at his Time and Pleasure: This was the Consolation given her Husband, from yours,

A. C.

About half an Hour after he had received this Letter, a Neighbour came, and with great Concern told me how much it grieved the Neighbourhood in general, to hear this Hero declare aloud in the open Street, that he could freely forgive my Husband, but swore to be the Destruction of the Bitch, his Wife. In which, answered I, he fulfils that Portion of Scripture, "A good Tree cannot bring forth bad Fruit; neither can a corrupt Tree bring forth good Fruit." Hence the Tree is known by its Fruit, for it is not the Advantage of a liberal Education, nor the Improvements of four Years Travel in *France* and *Rome*; neither the Benefits that he received from the Touch, nor the great Rise to a plentiful Fortune, that can make a corrupt Tree bring forth good Fruit: Cannot any Ass bray in the Streets? Nay, an Ideot can shout out, Bitch!

Great was his Industry in shewing this infamous Letter to Gentlemen, but not meeting with his desired Success, put him to the Torture, that Tyrants without Power feeleth. We having most of the Council that rode the Circuit with the Judges, my Husband went to *Newcastle* every Year to receive their Orders; and notwithstanding this infamous Letter, was resolved to go according to his Custom: But his Antagonist, although a Gentleman of Fortune, with his Lady, and Equipage, came but to his House the Evening before from *Northamptonshire*; yet these grand Visitors could not sooth the Venom of this savage Breast; for he left his Strangers to pursue his Revenge, and did compleat his Work. When my Husband spoke to the Chancellor, he was answered with Rogue, and Villain. Sir, said my

Husband,

Husband, I am neither; nor can I think my Antagonist will in cool Blood asperse me. Thou liest, answered the Chancellor, for I have been with this Gentleman this Instant, who hath convinced me of thy Vility; neither shall a Lawyer come to thy House, nor Judge, if I can keep them from it.

Yet for all these Threatenings, my Husband conscious of his Innocence, which he resolved to plead to the Council, in Hopes to find more Candour from them, but Rogue, Villain, and Beggar, were all their Answers. Notwithstanding this general Reproach, his guiltless Soul prompt him to see the Extent of this Malice. Accordingly he went to' know the Judges Will and Pleasure, and asking the Man that calls the Trials whether his Lords would be at his House, or not. The Man answered, Did they lodge at thy House last Year? My Husband answered, they did. Then, said he, I have heard of thy Fame, and we will all surely be at thy House; but as no Doubt thou hast some Business to transact, come to the Court after; then will I speak to my Lord, and there thou shalt receive thy Orders.

My Husband accordingly went to the Court, and one of the Bailiffs told the Crier that the Landlord waited his Answer. Let him stand up on high by me, answered the Crier, that all the Court may see him, and hear his Answer, which may add to the Credit of his House. My Husband said, I rather chuse to stand where I am. Then did the Crier mock my Husband, and with a loud Voice said, How durst thou, that is a Rogue! presume to ask the Judges to come to thy House? Dost thou not know that they come to hang Rogues, and not to encourage them: Behold the Impudence of this Landlord! that after he robbed the Council of their
Wine,

Wine, dare prefume to ask the Judges to lodge in
thy Houfe.

But four principal Inhabitants being in the Court,
in a Whifper faid, Behold the Extent, of inveterate
Malice; let us rebuke that Fellow, and do our
Neighbour Juftice. A worthy Gentleman of Integrity and Honour ftood up, and faid unto him, You
are taking a Liberty with that Man that very ill
becomes you, for we have heard that Story before
now, and believes him to be an honeft Man. Another faid, We that are his Neighbours, muft know
him better than thou that is a Stranger. A third
faid, He keeps the beft Houfe of Entertainment
and Cuftom in the Place. Which put this Fellow
to Silence.

This was two Affizes, and at the third there was
Debates between the Chancellor and Lawyer *Askew*,
who faid, he blamed *Cook* at the firft Hearing, but
his Acccufer at the fecond. He came to the Houfe,
and told us, that our great Adverfary had not fuc-
ceeded in his Undertaking againft us.

This Hero, ftill eager of Revenge, got to be a
Commiffioner of the Land Tax, and got fome of
his Allies in at the fame Time, I having all except
two of the old Commiffioners, and the Clerk,
that were all very worthy Guefts to my Houfe,
and fome of them much more powerful than himfelf: Although this Hero was the youngeft in the
Commiffion, yet in Expectation of having that Refpect paid him that was paid a Chairman, told
the Bench, that he had ordered a Dinner at an
Inn, where he hoped they all would dine with
him. But Mr. *Read* of *Chipchafe* anfwered, that it
was a Compliment paid the Judge at the General
Seffions, but as the Majority of the Commiffioners
of the Land Tax was Guefts to *Cook*, he had ordered

ed Dinner there. This, no doubt, was a hard Pill for this Hero to digeſt.

In 14 Days the Commiſſioners had another Meeting, and one of them came to me and ſaid, that the Chairman had made ſuch Propoſals as the Ties of Chriſtians obliged them to comply with, for, added he, this was his Speech. Gentlemen, as the rectifying the Land Tax on the Lands of *Roman* Catholicks requires our frequent Meetings, it muſt be very reſonable for us all dining together, as we may tranſact Buſineſs at that Time, in the Houſe where we dine; and is it not very hard for all to go to one Houſe? and I hope this worthy Aſſembly will oblige me in this Propoſal of good Neighbourhood, and Chriſtian Charity. But, added the Commiſſioner, I anſwered, that we had beſpoke Dinner at your Houſe this Day, and if he would dine with us, I would, if all the Reſt of your Gueſts joined with me, oblige him in this Propoſal: But what think you of it? I anſwered, that my Antagoniſt was ſeeming kind to his Neighbours: But would it not be more generous were it at his own Expence? for at that Rate he would but give me the fifth Part of my Trade, and at the ſame Time ſets himſelf out for the good Neighbour, although it ſeems as juſt for me to ſay, Why ſhould he have ſo much Land, and I none? or, Should not there be a Diſtribution of all Lands, and give each an equal Share? He ſaid, that I was certainly right; yet as they had promiſed him; they all reſolved to be the ſame Friends to our Houſe, as they were very certain they would not meet with better Entertainment, and I will let him know this, if he dines with us this Day, according to his Promiſe.

But he did not dine with them, nor ſent any Apology for the Breach of his Promiſe; yet they all went with this Hero to dine as they had promiſed him

him, and their Charges were three Half-crowns
each. This Gentleman addressing himself to the
Chairman, said, Sir, we have performed our Pro-
mise in attending you, as you proposed the last
Meeting, wherein you alledged, that it was hard
for all to go to one House; but here I plainly see
double the Number of Company that was at our
House, as every House hath its separate Custom,
and it appears to me that you would by Stratagem
take all the Custom from our House; although
you promised to dine with us, you did not, so I
hope you will not expect us being any longer at
your Call, for in obliging you we must hurt your
Neighbour.

Sir, answered I, my Creditors, and numerous Family of Children, requires the full Extent of my
Trade, which, contrary to the Laws of God and
Man, this Tyrant has made it his Business to obstruct. Now I begin to pity his poor ignoble Soul,
and wants to be free of his Malice: If I can meet
with a convenient House out of his Jurisdiction,
where I can receive the Profit of my Diligence and
Pains, and have a Prospect to live in Peace, I would
freely leave him the Field.

Two of the neighbouring Landlords making a
great Complaint of the Decay of Trade: Besides,
added they, we have not had Horse Races these
four Years, nor will the great Esquire let a Race
be as long as you are in the Town. I answered,
You two are both his Cousins by your Wives, and
if you can act the Part of two Politicians, I can put
you into the Way to trick Horse Races out of
him. They promised me they would. Then, answered I, go both of you to your great Cousin,
and footh his vain Glory with reverend Bows, and
tell him how much you are piqued that my Husband hath had 16 *l.* of the Booking Money of the

laſt Races four Years, and braves you, by ſaying, that he never will pay it up, till you bring him a Lift, ſigned with the Eſquire's Name for another Race, then you ſhall receive the Money, and not before.

Accordingly they went, were received with a hearty Welcome, and bid them come in the Evening, and ſhou!d have their Requeſts fulfilled : But, added he, my Steward, ſhall receive the Money. Very well, ſaid I, leave that Part for me to act : But firſt I'll lend you the Parchment that they ſubſcribe their Names in. But, anſwered they, take Care not to raiſe his Spleen againſt us. Leave that to me alſo.

In the Evening comes the two Landlords, and their great Couſin's Steward, who ſaid, that he came to receive the Booking Money that we had, which was to help up the Races. What Races? ſaid I. One of the Landlords anſwered, Your Huſband ſaid, that at the Receipt of theſe Gentlemens Names to another Race, he would pay up that Money. But where is their Names, ſaid I. So he gave me the Lift, I read it, and ſaid, Is not this the very Parchment that I bought laſt Year, and you were refuſed ſigning it? We know the Parchment to be yours, but you have no Right to theſe Gentlemens Names. I will diſpute that Right with you, or your grand Maſter, ſaid I, turning to the Steward : Theſe two Fellows have been with your heroick Maſter, ſcheming and contriving to get this Booking Money into thy Maſter's Coffer, or ſtrong Box we will call it; but ask him what Right he hath to make this Demand. Theſe Fellows had only my Husband's Promiſe for the Money, which Promiſe they reſigned to thy Maſter; but I don't think that it would be doing the Sportſmen Juſtice, to give this Money out of my Husband's Hand,

for

for befides we fhall make great Advantage in trading with it, fo that putting it into your Mafter's ftrong Box, where there is no Need of it, is burying this Talent in the Earth: Therefore tell your Mafter, that I treat for Peace with him, as well for his own Sake as mine, that he may enjoy his plentiful Fortune with Pleafure, and that I may reap the Profit of my lawful Induftry, without his Interruption.

But inftead of this Hero adhereing to my Treaty of Peace, open War was declared againft me, nor fhould there be any Races; yet as we had his Name fubfcribed, the Gentlemen feemed all well pleafed with the Stratagem, and with Pleafure fubfcribed to the Races.————The Ladies told me, that if I could get a Room fit for an Affembly, they would come and make up the Lofs that I had fuftained by my envious Enemy: I having a worthy Landlord, told him the Ladies Requeft, who with great Pleafure was at the Charge of pulling down a Partition, which made a Room 13 Yards long, having five Safh-windows, made it a commodious Affembly-room, painted all the Doors and Windows, and the Ballifters of the Stairs; during which Time my Antagonift was taking great Pains to difannul the Races, told the Gentlemen, that it was fo late on the Year, by the Indolence of thofe Fellows, that there could be no Races. But the Gentlemen faid, that it would be a very good Time for them, befides they were all defirous of fome Sport, it being fo long fince they had any: And, added they, Mrs. *Cook* hath got a long Room for an Affembly, fo that we fhall get a Dance.

But Sir *John Cope*'s Army and the *Highlanders* being very near each other in *Scotland*, gave great Confufion, and a great Meeting of Gentlemen being

ing called together at *Morpeth*, this Hero stood up, and told the Audience, that the People in *Hexham*, contrary to his Inclination, would have Horse Races, which might give a great many Papists and Jacobites an Opportunity of meeting, who might conspire together at this critical Juncture: He therefore thought it requisite and necessary to have the Bench to make an Order to forbid these Races, for the Nation's Safety. A noble Baronet answered, Sir, Races in such little Towns are made for the Benefit of low Life People, instead of suppressing them, let us all unanimously meet, and spend some Money, to help them to live.

But this did not answer the Hero's End, for whether he got an Order signed by the Bench of Justices or not, he came Home, sent for the two Landlords and my Husband, and said to them, You all know the Confusion the Nation is in, with the Rebels in *Scotland*, and their Defeat over the King's Army, which put the whole Nation into such a Ferment, as the Bench thought proper to make an Order to forbid Races, and to deem them Rebels that presumed to let a Race be on *Tyne Green*. To which my Husband answered, that these Races were advertised by the Royal Order, the Horses were all booked according to that Advertisement, and if his Worship would satisfy these Men, he was willing, but not otherwise.

He bid him send them to him, which my Husband did, and they returned with an Order from this Hero to my Husband, to return the Jockeys their Booking Money, and to pay each Man two Guineas. He told them their Booking Money they should have, but must get their Charges from this Hero: They went and told him their Answer; who then sent an Attorney to my Husband to tell him, that if he would not pay the Jockeys that Money, he would commit him to Goal. He anſwered, that he was willing to go there by his Mittimuſs; but tell him, he ſhall either pay the Jockeys, or there ſhall be Races.——— Every Man came with two Guineas, there being 11 Horſes booked, and Revenge coſt 22 Guineas, rather than we ſhould have any Advantage by theſe Races.

The Landlord of the Queen's Head, in *Morpeth*, died then, ſo my Husband went and took that Houſe, Furniture, and Stock: The Landlord of the Houſe gave Bond with my Husband for the Money, which was 369 *l.* We were obliged to keep the Inn at *Hexham* three Months longer, ſo that we had both theſe Inns in theſe Confuſions: The King's Army being at *Hexham*, the two *Dutch* Generals were both at our Houſe, when my Daughter had it to manage, which ſhe did to the Admiration of all that ſaw her; for ſhe was but 17 Years of Age, and dreſt above 60 Diſhes of Meat every Day, for five Days; nor did ſhe get any Reſt at Night, but what ſhe got in the Kitchen.

My youngeſt Daughter came to me at *Morpeth*, and ſaid, that ſhe had rather die than ſee another Camp at *Hexham*; although, ſaid ſhe, I had much the better of my Siſter, that never had her Cloaths off for five Days: The two *Dutch* Cooks made nothing for the Generals but Soops, and my poor Siſter, with the Help that I could make, had all the Meat to dreſs, and my Father and her ſlept in the Kitchen, amongſt 50 military Men. We were all thankful you were not there, for the Severity of the Weather, Hurry, and Confuſion, would have killed you.

For

For I had not recovered of a Miscarriage, which very much impaired my Health, and reduced me to great Weakness; yet in this bad State of Health I had more Cookery to perform than I had at *Hexham*, for the Army came all through *Morpeth* for *Scotland*, I generally had 50 Soldiers billeted on my House, and had moft of the Officers that came from *Hexham*. I as frequently had 14 Officers as 50 Men, befides the Servants, and none but my younger Daughter to help me to drefs all the Meat for fuch a numerous Family. But how to order fo very great a Family at this Time, and pleafe all Parties was the Query: The long March from *Hexham* to *Morpeth* (25 Miles) in a Storm, fatigued the poor Soldiers greatly, and after thefe long Marches had no Beds but Straw, fome lay in Barns without any Fire; but I refolved to make my Share of them as happy as I could, for every Day I boiled two Stone of Pork, one Stone of Beef, and half a Peck of Peafe, and made 20 Gallons of Porrage, with Plenty of Barley, Roots, and Leaks in them. I told them, that that was all the Attendance they would get, having fo many of their Officers to provide for; nor would they get any Breakfaft or Supper, for I would take none of their Money: This was not only my Duty, but my Intereft, for I had not the Trouble of making them Supper, nor Breakfaft, which would coft me all the Money I fhould receive from them, exclufive of their Dinners.

After I had got this great Hurry over, the Army paft, and got my Houfe into Order, I had a Vifit from my Landlord, who told me, that a Coufin of his came, and told him that he muft come to her Houfe, as there was fomething of Importance to communicate to him: When I came there, faid he, I was very much upbraided with two great Coufins
of

of mine, the Aunt and her Nephew. She told me how much I had leffened their Family, in letting this Houfe to fuch a Rogue as you, for which Offence it would be incurring their Difpleafure for ever. I anfwered the Landlord, that I was very forry that he fhould meet with any Infult upon my Account, but more that he fhould be related to thefe two troublefome Adverfaries of mine; for, added I, I have left one of the beft of Neighbourhoods, to get rid of them, and live in Tranquillity, having undergone fix Years Perfecution, three Years of which ftands in Record, well attefted by all the Council, that rides the *Northern* Circuit, and moft of the Gentry in the County.

He anfwered, that it was his Belief, that his Coufin would in a very little Time, be the brighteft Gentleman in the County. He muft improve very faft in Perfon, Mind, and Fortune then, anfwered I, for he has at prefent many Superiors in all thefe Talents.

When the Duke of *Cumberland* came through *Morpeth*, after the Battle of *Culloden*, all the grand Gentry in the County affembled at *Morpeth*, in Hopes of feeing his Royal Highnefs, to congratulate him on the Victory: A fumptuous Entertainment was provided on that Occafion, and when all Souls were filled with Joy, his was brimful of the old Caufe, fo full that he burft forth to the Audience, and faid, that *Cook* was a Rebel! a Rogue! a Villain!! But a certain Gentleman reproved him at that Inftant, and bid him fpeak with more Candour, for *Cook* had the Character of a harmlefs honeft Man; neither was he meddlefome in State Affairs.

I re-

I returned this Gentleman my humbleſt Thanks, and ſaid, that I had great Reaſon to ſuſpect him for intending to make ſuch an Information to his Royal Highneſs, that there might be an Order to plunder all Jacobites; for I was privately informed that there was to be a Plunder, and our Houſe was to be the firſt. But as his Royal Highneſs made ſo ſhort a Stop we were not moleſted.——The next News was, that he would ſtand Candidate for Parliament Man for the County: Then, ſaid I, he cannot keep the Freeholders from my Houſe. A great Number of them coming one Day, Billets were brought to them, for ſuch Houſes as were told them, but they rejected the Billets.

When the Bills were paid, my Hero's Steward brought in the 22 Guineas that his Maſter paid the Jockeys; but my Husband produced a Receipt for eight Guineas of this Money, that was paid by the Orders of four Gentlemen Subſcribers: So my Huſband told the Steward that he was prepared for their Objection to his Bill; but as he had all his ſeparate Bills atteſted by the Freeholders, who ſaid, that if his Bills were objected, they would pay him themſelves. The Steward peruſing theſe Bills, ſaid, You may very juſtly demand your Money, for, in my Opinion, it exceeds all the Parlimentearing Bills for Juſtice. The Steward accordingly paid him the 50 l.

There was a grand Meeting of Gentry at *Morpeth* Races, and I had Orders at Seven o'Clock, to provide Supper for 20 Ladies and Gentlemen, to be ready preciſely at Eight. I never having ſuch an Order before, rouſed up the Mettle of the whole Houſe, and had every Thing in Order to receive this grand Company, amongſt whom was this Hero, his Lady, and Aunt.

'This

This Supper pleafed fo well, that four noble E-
fquires befpoke a Dinner for 40 Ladies and Gentlemen, and ordered a long Table to be made, to
reach from one End of the Room to the other. I
received this Order with Joy, and had the cold Table finifhed, when I received a Meffage, that this
Hero had begged it as the greateft Favour, that the
Ladies and Gentlemen would dine with him at the
Black Bull. However, I had as many Gentlemen,
and Servants, as eat up my Dinner.

My eldeft Daughter marrying a young Man, who
had an Eftate at the Deceafe of an old Aunt: There
being an Inn advertifed to be lett at *Newcaftle*, my
Son went with me and took the Houfe, which my
Daughter and I got very decently furnifhed; I did
as much as I was able, and no more, and what all
Parents do for hopeful Children, according to their
Abilities.

This was no fooner done than a Rumour arofe
that *Cook* was broke, there being a Bond and Judgment entered againft him for 730 *l.* and that his
Wife had fet up her Daughter out of the Creditors
Goods: The Highways were befet with People to
inform Travellers, and his Guefts went paft his
Houfe. The Creditors upbraided him with the Injuftice he had treated them with, and he pleaded
his Innocence: They faid, It is the fame Defraud,
if you connived with your Wife; befides you have
a Judgment of 730 *l.* which is entered againft you.
He told them, that he never was asked a Judgment
but by the Landlord of the Houfe, who was bound
for 369 *l.* 320 *l.* of which is paid: Neither, added
he, did I give him Judgment, for he faid he wanted no more but a Letter of an Attorney.

The

The Landlord's Nephew came to my Husband next Day, and said, that notwithstanding all the Rumour, there was no Judgment entered, and if he would sign a Bond of Release of Errors, it would save him 4 l. Charge. Villain! said my Husband, hast thou bit me once, and would bite me again. And flew into such a Fury, that if the Fellow had not absconded, he would have threshed him as the Villain deserved; yet this Repulse did not hinder the Fellow to watch a favourable Opportunity in my Husband's Absence, of soliciting me to persuade my Husband, for the Sake of my numerous Family, to sign this Bond of Release of Errors, which will save 4 l. Charge. I answered, that I never heard of such a Bond, nor did I know of a Judgment: It appears to me that you durst not venture to execute it, nor enter upon the Spoil, without this Bond of Release of Errors.

What, answered he, do you suspect my great Cousin to be at the Bottom of this? Thou must know that best, Fellow! said I: He came to Town Yesterday, was invisible two Hours, in which Time it may be presumed he hath given thou thy Instructions. No doubt but he has promised thou a Reward, besides the Plunder of our House; but if thou fail of getting this Bond of Release of Errors executed, his envious Soul will curse thou for thy Botchery, in not inserting this Bond of Release of Errors in the Bond and Judgment, which might have saved thy Cousin a Counsel's Fee, who, no doubt, would tell him, that if his Attorney had known his Business, he would have done it effectually at first.

This being the first Job of Consequence that thou hast been employed in since thou got out

of

of *Fleet* Prison, after thou had gotten 1500 *l*. out of the Country, gave thy Father a Bond and Judgment of 400 *l*. who entered and sold thy Goods and Chattels, took Home thy Wife, that has been a secret Paunbroker ever since: Thou did not go into *Fleet* Prison, to wait an Act of Grace, without Provision; nor has any visible Way of getting Bread, has very little Sence, yet with that small Matter has done much Harm; for thy Brother in Law, after the Judge had given a Charge to the Jury, told them that if they found a Verdict for *Cook*, it would bring Actions against all Corn-sellers: This Fellow! (thy Brother in Law) was so industrious in telling the Jury, although he was three Times forbid the Room; he gained his Point, they brought a Verdict for the Villain that sold us a Sample of good Corn, and brought in the Stock bad rotten Corn, which we never would take Possession of, and although the Judge turned the Jury back, they brought in the same Verdict. The Corn and Trial cost us 70 *l*. whether thy envious Cousin was the Prompter in this hellish Scheme, the Devil and thou knows best; for such Envy, Hatred, and Malice, renders you the Seed of *Beelzebub*: Thou knows thyself guilty of Forgery, for which a Halter is thy Desart; thy Cousin is a rich Rogue, thou art a very poor Rogue, and a great Fool, almost a naked Beggar, waiting on Help from thy covetous Uncle, who can part with nothing in his Life, nor will thou get ony of his Riches at his Death: I am an excellent Fortune-teller, that will do my Creditors so much Justice, as to keep such a ravenous Wolf as thou art, from devouring what is theirs. Tell this Cousin of thine, that he hath made many Trials, but will be victorious at last; yet, I can brave him with what very few of his Kindred possesses, and that is an honest Soul! a Treasure that can soar above the Malice of Tyrants; whose Judge can frustrate all treacherous Designs.

Away

Away goes this Mifcreant, and immediately comes
his Wife, to know what Conference I had with
her Husband, that had deprived him of his Speech.
What can be the Matter? faid I. Is it a Sting of
Confcience, or a Difappointment of Releafe of Errors. At which Words fhe burft into Tears, and
faid, It hath been my hard Fate, to be matched to
a Man without Senfe, or Morals; this the Judgment makes manifeft, done to fo good a Friend as
you have been in our Diftrefs: Thefe Tears can
witnefs the Sincerty of a grateful Soul, to difcharge
all Obligations that I ftand indebted to you, fign
this Bond.

Aloud I laugh'd, and faid, You are two Creatures,
That differs not in Minds, but much in Features:
Prevaricator, up thy Tears dry,
That Bond cannot be figned, the Reafon why,
I muft my Husband's Hand from Paper keep,
Left ye two laugh, while we two both fhould weep.

And bid her go Home to bewail the Hardfhips of
her difconfolate Mourner, without Senfe or Morals.

Then did I fend for the Landlord, and the two
Gentlemen that were Truftees to the Will of the
deceafed Landlord: They produced the Bond, and
received 30 *l.* which was all their Demands. Then,
faid I, Sir, this 30 *l.* was all the Money you could
have any Pretence of entering a Judgment of 730 *l.*
which Bond you have no further Pretence to keep.
He delivered up this Bond, as ftrong as my Hufband could be made Debter for 369 *l.* and to pay
five *per Cent.* Intereft. I read the Bond to thefe
Gentlemen, and faid to the Landlord, Sir, if you
were a Chriftian, you durft not have fleep'd a Night
in your Bed with this Bond, from a Man that never
received your Money; and had you taken a Bond
of

of Indemnity of that Bond, why was it not mentioned in this? Befides you fwore not to take a
Bond and Judgment. He anfwered, that it was as
much againft his Inclination to do it, as to tear the
Flefh from his Bones, but he was put upon it. I
know your Prompter, faid I.

This Artifice tript up the Trade, I could not anfwer Credit, and plainly faw the Fruits of my hard
Labour demolifh every Day, and what was the greateft Hardfhip, I under the Cenfure of defrauding the
Creditors, and the Reproach of all cenforious Mifcreants; my Friends looked cold on me, fo that I
had only the Confolation of an honeft Heart to con-
dole with. I pleaded with the Creditors for Time,
and fold 200 *l.* Worth of Furniture, and took a
Houfe on the *Keyfide, Newcaftle*: When I furnifhed my Houfe, I propofed keeping a Paftry Cook
Shop, befides felling Malt Liquor, Wine, and Spirits, and got 2000 Gallons of Malt Liquor brewed.
Within a Month after we left *Morpeth*, my Hufband was feized for 30 *l.* by a Malfter, and as I had
paid up all the Money to the Creditors, I could
not releafe my Husband from the Bailiffs. In this
Diftrefs I fent for a Wine Merchant, to whom we
owed 20 *l.* and told my Hardfhips. But his Countenance faid, he had rather I paid this Bill; adding
that he had Notice given him, before we left
Morpeth, that if he fhould give us any Credit
he would never receive Two-pence, as there was
Judgment againft you for 700 *l.* But, Sir, anfwered I, did we not balance with you, fince you
got this Notice? and paid 300 *l.* and can fhew you
that Bond of 730 *l.* with all the Charges of entering
this Judgment, and a Receipt in full of all Accompts
concerning this Bond, from the Man that took that
Advantage of my Husband, in order to break his
Credit, who did not receive a Farthing from him:
So can I fhew you Receipts from my Creditors for
10,000 *l.*

10,000 *l*. paid honeftly; all the Demands the World can make upon us is 380 *l*. and we have as much as may pay 10 *s*. to the Pound, after ten Years Perfecution. The Creditors had a Meeting, on the Notice, that was given from this Wine Merchant; but thefe Propofals were not accepted, nor would they offer any Terms but Contempt; in fhort, I then became the Scorn of wealthy Fools.

I could tell you fuch a Story, as would force Tears from your Eyes; but I rather chufe to rejoice at the flowery Paths you have travelled in, then fee you mourn at the Briars and Thorns I have had to brufh through, purfued by Wolves and Bears in human Shapes: If you live to read the Hiftory of my Life, in it you perhaps may fee fomething deferving the Prefs. For although I never was out of the Counties of *Durham* and *Northumberland* but 10 Days, and found 30 Years fo hard travelling in the latter, as may let the World fee what Providence hath enabled one Mortal to undergo.

Who does me wrong, or hurts my Reputation,
If to my Judge I make true Application,
His Wifdom, Goodnefs, fupreme Excellence,
Aids and affifts in clearing Innocence:
A Tyrant that works hard to hurt his Neighbour,
Deferves a juft Reward for all his Labour.

F I N I S.

You may also be interested in these titles:

Townsends is please to make available a growing list of rare and valuable books from the 18th and early 19th centuries, including those listed below. Be sure to visit our website for a complete list of titles.

Cookbooks

The Art of Cookery by Hannah Glasse (1765)

The Domestick Coffee-Man by Humphrey Broadbent (1722) and *The New Art of Brewing Beer* by Thomas Tyron (1690)

The Complete Housewife by Eliza Smith (1730)

The Universal Cook by John Townshend (1773)

The Practice of Cookery by Mrs. Frazer (1791 & 1795)

The London Art of Cookery by John Farley (1787)

The Complete Confectioner by Hannah Glasse (1765)

A New and Easy Method of Cookery by Elizabeth Cleland (1755)

The English Art of Cookery by Richard Briggs (1788)

18th & Early 19th-Century Brewing by multiple authors

The Lady's Assistant by Charlotte Mason (1777)

The Experienced English Housekeeper by Elizabeth Raffald (1769)

The Professed Cook by B. Clermont (1769)

The Cook's and Confectioner's Dictionary by John Nott (1723)

The Modern Art of Cookery Improved by Ann Shackleford (1765)

The Country Housewife's Family Companion by William Ellis (1750)

A Collection of Above Three Hundred Receipts by Mary Kettelby (1714)

England's Newest Way in All Sorts of Cookery by Henry Howard (1726)

—*····※·····*—

Biographies & Journals

The Hessians by multiple authors

Travels Through the Interior Parts of North-America in the Years 1766, 1767, and 1768 by Jonathan Carver (1778)

The Women of the American Revolution, Volumes 1, 2, & 3 by Elizabeth Ellet (1848)

The Backwoods of Canada by Catharine Parr Traill (1836)

Travels into North America by Peter Kalm (1760)

New Travels in the United States of America. Performed in 1788 and *The Commerce of America and Europe* by J.P. Brissot De Warville (1792 & 1795)

The Journal of Nicholas Cresswell, 1774–1777 by Nicholas Cresswell (1924)

An Account of the Life of the Late Reverend Mr. David Brainerd by Jonathan Edwards (1765 & 1824)

Travels for Four Years and a Half in the United States of America During 1798, 1799, 1800, 1801, and 1802 by John Davis (1909)

Travels through North and South Carolina, Georgia, East and West Florida by William Bartram (1792)

A Tour in the United States of America, Volumes 1 & 2 by John F. Smyth Stuart (1784)

Simcoe's Military Journal by J. G. Simcoe (1844)

—*''''☆''''*—

Townsends

www.townsends.us

Made in the USA
Columbia, SC
20 September 2018